'I believe that Anna Ashby's important book is destined to become a classic and *the* signature book on Restorative Yoga. A much-needed guide in this age of chaos and stress.'

– Max Strom, author of A life Worth Breathing, *3x TEDx speaker and global teacher of yoga and healing breathing patterns*

'This considered book is a timely reminder that the essence of yoga is by definition restorative. Anna Ashby's years of practice and teaching reflected in her inspired writing, not only point the way to a profoundly authentic yoga experience, but make you want to get out the props and accept her invitation there and then. A valuable contribution to the profession.'

– John Stirk, author of The Original Body: Primal Movement for Yoga teachers *and* Deeper Still: Authentic Embodiment for Yoga Teachers

'Anna is one of my favourite teachers of all time. She is a teacher's teacher and has the ability to keep things simple and straight talking. It was in her Restorative classes that I had the "Restorative light-bulb moment". As I have gotten older, having a Restorative practice and a meditation practice has been essential to my mental and physical self-care practice. Anna has the ability to explain the benefits of the Restorative practice and how important it is to pay attention to the nervous system in such a way that you shift your perspective. We have spent our lifetime learning how important "doing" is. Anna is reminding us of the importance of "being".'

– Nadia Narain, co-author of the bestselling book Self-Care for the Real World

'Anna Ashby's approach to Restorative practice reflects not only her years of practice, but the nuance and wisdom she brings to everything she teaches. Highly recommended.'

– Sally Kempton, author of Meditation for the Love of It *and* Awakening Shakti

'Relaxation and alertness together are the axis in which a joyful, peaceful and compassionate life spins. How does one refine the ability to drop into this combined state of being? This is the task Anna has taken on in *Restorative Yoga* and she has succeeded profoundly. She answers the why and the how and leaves us with a practice manual essential for everyday sanity and health.'

- Rodney Yee, international yoga teacher and co-director of Urban Zen Integrative Therapy (UZIT)

D1496390

of related interest

Yoga Therapy for Insomnia and Sleep Recovery
An Integrated Approach to Supporting Healthy Sleep and Sustaining Energy All Day
Lisa Sanfilippo
ISBN 978 1 84819 391 8
eISBN 978 0 85701 348 4

Restorative Yoga for Ethnic and Race-Based Stress and Trauma
Gail Parker
Forewords by Octavia F. Raheem and Amy Wheeler
Illustrated by Justine Ross
ISBN 978 1 78775 185 9
eISBN 978 1 78775 186 6

Transforming Ethnic and Race-Based Traumatic Stress with Yoga
Gail Parker
Illustrated by Justine Ross
ISBN 978 1 78775 753 0
eISBN 978 1 78775 754 7

Restoring Prana
A Therapeutic Guide to Pranayama and Healing Through the Breath for
Yoga Therapists, Yoga Teachers, and Healthcare Practitioners
Robin L. Rothenberg
Foreword by Richard Miller
Illustrated by Kirsteen Wright

RESTORATIVE YOGA

Power, Presence and Practice for Teachers and Trainees

Anna Ashby

Foreword by Richard Rosen
Illustrations by Sarah J. Coleman
Photography by Karen Yeomans

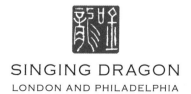

SINGING DRAGON
LONDON AND PHILADELPHIA

First published in Great Britain in 2022 by Singing Dragon
An imprint of Jessica Kingsley Publishers
An imprint of Hodder & Stoughton Ltd
An Hachette Company

1

A CIP catalogue record for this title is available from the
British Library and the Library of Congress

ISBN 978 1 78775 739 4
eISBN 978 1 78775 740 0

Printed and bound in Great Britain by Bell & Bain Limited

Jessica Kingsley Publishers' policy is to use papers that are natural, renewable and recyclable
products and made from wood grown in sustainable forests. The logging and manufacturing
processes are expected to conform to the environmental regulations of the country of origin.

Jessica Kingsley Publishers
Carmelite House
50 Victoria Embankment
London EC4Y 0DZ

www.singingdragon.com

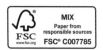

Permissions

Jackie Morris for *The Unwinding and Other Dreamings*

Bill Mahony for his translations of *Taittirīya Upaniṣad*

Models in photos: Yvonne O'Garro and Sherman Sam

Shared experiences of Restorative Yoga: Andy Beyst, Felicity Daly, Jodie Jackson, Joyce McMiken, Malcolm Stern, Sarah Deco and Yvonne O'Garro

To my mother – source, sustenance and role model extraordinaire

and

To the yoga practices and teachings that nourish and guide

Power

Become still and turn inwards.
Supported and safe, be at ease.
Rest and heal.
Experience the aliveness within.
Awaken
to Fullness of Being.

Presence

Experience the moment
as it unfolds;
Soft, abiding fullness.
Where self meets Self
And merges
in ecstasy.
An ever-present Joy.

Practice

Feel into, sense and know,
inner being as
Sanctuary;
Discipline,
a wellspring that liberates.
Turn inwards and…
Listen.

Contents

PART II: PRESENCE

PART III: PRACTICE

Foreword

Much like the Hatha Yoga we in the West practise today, Restorative Yoga is both very old and very new. It has a humble beginning. 'Lie on your back on the ground like a corpse,' wrote the yogi Swātmārāma in the *Haṭhapradīpikā* ('Light on Hatha Yoga'), slightly more than 500 years ago. 'This is *śavāsana*, the Corpse pose. It does away with fatigue and brings rest to your conscious mind' (1.32). To us, accustomed as we are to our teacher's detailed instructions, Swātmārāma barely skims the surface. But we should remember these old texts were more like summaries or outlines of the teaching; the specifics on how to put that teaching into play were passed by word of mouth from the guru to the student.

Nonetheless, in Swātmārāma's two brief sentences we see the rudiments, the how and why, of our modern Restorative practice: we're to lie supine 'on the ground' (the most stable and secure of all positions) and maintain a corpse-like stillness (which has a corresponding effect on the brain) that promises to re-invigorate the body and calm the mind. Over the 400 years following the *Haṭhapradīpikā*, in the dozen or so texts I searched, the written instruction for the pose stays pretty much the same. 'Lie down on the floor like a corpse,' reads the mid-19th-century *Śrītattvanidhi* ('Blessed Treasure of Reality'), 'this is *śavāsana*' (70). Also, during this same time, Corpse is apparently used mostly, if not exclusively, to put the finishing touch on an *āsana* practice.

This all begins to change in the early decades of the 20th century, where several factors contribute to the emergence of Restorative Yoga. There's the re-invention and popularization of Hatha Yoga by certain Indian teachers, and the gradual westward migration of this re-vitalized practice, especially after the 1960s. With the slow but steady increase of newly minted yogis, and the consequent impracticality of face-to-face meetings with a guru for teaching, there appear for the first time full-blown instruction manuals, written not for the ascetic as were the old texts, but for the general public for whom yoga was a part, either great or small, but not the be all and end all of their lives. These books then needed to be far more expansive than the old texts. We see, for example, in Yogācarya Sundaram's *The Secret of Happiness or Yogic Physical Culture* (1928, p.85), that Corpse is covered in a six-page essay that offers directions not only on how to enter the pose, but what to do while in it and how to properly exit. 'One should not get up suddenly or jerk into position immediately after *śavāsana*.' Sound familiar?

There's also a recognition that Corpse needn't be limited to the finish of an *āsana* practice; that its soothing effects could be beneficial in many different everyday situations. So Shri Yogendra, founder of the Yoga Institute of India, writes in his *Yoga Asanas Simplified* (1928, p.158): 'Whenever physical or mental fatigue is experienced or the mind is agitated, the practice of *śavāsana*…is recommended.' Note the opening word, 'whenever'.

Finally, it was during this time that science-minded researchers like Swami Kuvalayananda, founder of the Kaivalyadhama Health and Yoga Research Center, used instruments like x-rays and spirometers to measure the effects of the various practices on test subjects. So we find, for example, in the July 1926 (pp.229–232) issue of Kuvalayananda's quarterly house organ, *Yoga-Mimamsa*, a four-page report on Corpse, in which it's broken down into three stages, with suggested cautions and points of study listed – a far cry from Swātmārāma.

All this sets the stage for the book you hold in your hands. I had the opportunity to witness from afar – 5300 miles or so, she in the UK, me in California – Anna's year-long writing journey, from the conception of this book to its completion. Like any project of this magnitude, as I can vouch from personal experience, it's been for her both a labour of love and a labour. The end result – and yes, I admit to being unreservedly biased – will surely become, in a very short while, a classic in its field.

I'd like to use the space I've been allotted here to explain why I think this book is so important, even ground breaking. It's no secret that we Westerners favour a vigorous practice. Witness the widespread popularity of flow-type classes, spin-offs all from that epitome of hyperactive yoga, the Pattabhi Jois-style Ashtanga Yoga. Most of us believe that in order to reach some goal, however ill defined, we need to make an effort; and certainly, this is in line with one of the two traditional 'wings' of yoga, *abhyāsa*, which may be rendered into English as consistent and persistent practice. What we don't favour is inactivity, what most of us think of as 'wasting time'. How is it possible to progress towards a goal by doing nothing?

So what we tend to forget, or ignore, is the other 'wing' of traditional yoga, without which, like a bird with only one wing, we figuratively can't get off the ground. This is *vairāgya*, a word usually translated as 'dispassion', and what I prefer to interpret as 'letting go', but only of those things in our life that detract from our health and happiness and lessen our compassion for others.

How can 'doing nothing' be considered part of a legitimate practice? How can it make our 'doing something' more effective and so – potentially at least, for in yoga there are never any guarantees – deliver us to our goal more quickly? I once had a teacher who always reminded us in class that there are many things we do to ourselves unconsciously, both physically and mentally, that restrict our movements and breath. Before we make the effort to change ourselves and move towards our goal, he advised us that we first have to be at least aware of those unknown obstacles, otherwise much of our practice will be self-defeating and, ironically, a waste of time. To become aware of those obstacles takes patience, persistence and, above all, stillness, which allows us to step back and observe ourselves from, I suppose we can say, a bird's eye view.

For Anna, this practice ideally results not only in the restoration of the body-mind, which could after all be just as easily accomplished with a nice nap. No, Anna's goal is two-fold and looks to transcend the practice's usual intent: first, the restoration of our missing wing, through the stillness that leads effortlessly to self-enquiry and the subsequent revelation and release of our unconscious 'doings'; and second, once we have both our wings intact, the restoration of our self, the ultimate source of health and happiness and compassion.

I think the one thing, if I had to choose, that I find most remarkable about this teaching is her integration of doing/non-doing in the very breath of our being. Ask most people about breathing and I wager they'll talk only about its doing – the inhales and exhales. But Anna assures us that the pauses, the non-doings, between these doings, are equally essential to our lives. In Chapter 8, The Breath as Teacher and Friend, there's a sub-section, 'The space in between', that being the pauses in the breath. Like the yogis of old, who heard in the sound of our breath our unbreakable connection to the Absolute, Anna sees the 'still points', silences between the sounds, as also 'little doorways into the infinite', through which we can pass to that 'seamless state of formless being, beyond objectification, which resonates as joy'.

Every now and again, when the occasion arises, I 'volunteer' to assist one of my yoga teacher friends in their classes. It's an experience I always find both educational and humbling, which doubles whenever I'm in London – which isn't often enough – and I assist Anna in one of her Restorative classes. I'm always so impressed with how smoothly the class proceeds, how well conceived is the sequence, how accessible for all levels of students are the poses, and how clearly and precisely she verbalizes the instructions. I could go on, about her expert adjustments and use of props, but I think you get the picture. Practising with this book is the closest you can come to a live class with Anna. All you need to make it as real as possible is to hear in your imagination the three chimes she makes with her Tibetan bells to signal the end of *śavāsana*, and her concluding Oms. I believe then you'll find yourself in the state yogis call by various names, *ānanda*, *harṣa*, *utsava*, or if you prefer, joy.

Richard Rosen

Acknowledgements

This book represents the input of many. It could not have happened without the two-way exchange of knowledge and goodwill between student and teacher, along with a collective wish to dive deep into the experience of human 'being'.

Many thanks to Singing Dragon for publishing this book and supporting yoga teachers in deepening their study and practice.

Thank you to my students, who have been a source of inspiration, and to triyoga in London, who gave me a home. I especially wish to thank Jonathan Sattin, who has always supported me and without whom I may not have walked down this path.

Thanks to family, friends, friends of friends, teachers and students, who have played an essential role in supporting the evolution of the book: Giorgos Alexandris, Andy Beyst, Calia Brencsons Van Dyk, Chloe Rose Campbell, Sarah Jane Coleman, Felicity Daly, Sarah Deco, Annette Dyvi, Kiki Felipe, Thea Foster, Jodie Jackson, Emma Lecoeur, Joyce McMiken, Yvonne O'Garro, Lauren Phillips, Catarina Portugal, Luciana Freire Rangel, Sherman Sam, Malcom Stern, Michael Stravato, Genny Wilkinson-Priest and Karen Yeomans.

A particular thanks to Ali Masterman, Lucy May Constantini and Sujata Ringawa for the generosity of their time and skill with editing.

I am very grateful for my teachers and teaching partners from whom I have learned so much over the years: David Behrens, Jason Birch, Gillian Evans, John Friend, Kevin Gardiner, Steve Haines, Jean Hall, Jacqueline Hargreaves, Bill Mahony, Joey Miles, Donald Moyer, Aki Omori, Jayne Orton, Carlos Pomeda, Richard Rosen, Daniel Simpson, Nikki Slade, Chris Swain and Tony Watson.

Thank you to James, the pillar of strength in my life.

A special thank you to my mum, who always lets me know what she thinks!

I'd like to extend my deep respect to the yoga tradition with its innumerable practitioners and teachers, who have preserved and passed on this extraordinary body of knowledge.

And finally, my deepest gratitude to the Siddha Yoga lineage and especially Gurumayi Chidvilasananda, who, with compassion and grace, has led me on a path of awakening, and who remains the inspiration for my life's endeavour.

Introduction

This book gives tangible form to the many years I've been practising and teaching Restorative Yoga. My intent in writing this book is to collate and share the different aspects of this style of yoga practice in order to help yoga teachers and practitioners from differing backgrounds, styles of yoga and other modalities to better understand, practise and incorporate its benefits.

Not only does the book offer the essential knowledge necessary for understanding the practice and its purpose, it also sheds light on the interrelationship between stress, the nervous system and how Restorative Yoga can serve as a means for re-establishing balance.

In addition, the book provides a helpful framework for enquiring into the experience of the practice, as well as considering the ways in which we may ourselves contribute to imbalance through unexamined cultural and societal attitudes towards work and living.

Especially when the perception of threat or uncertainty is high (I write this book at the time of the coronavirus pandemic), being able to recognize the signs of prolonged stress and understand how to support the nervous system when it is in 'overdrive' are key to maintaining good health and a sense of wellbeing.

Restorative Yoga offers a high-leverage, empowered practice for living well, particularly in times of adversity and distress. It offers a valuable means for managing fear, tension and stress levels through awareness and presence; it can also serve to reaffirm deeper aspirations with regard to yoga practice. By becoming still and aware, this style of practice offers a pathway to an experience of inner freedom through exploration and enquiry, releasing tension that frees the breath. It can teach us (if we let it) how to access inner joy and peacefulness, regardless of outer circumstances.

I started practising yoga in the San Francisco Bay Area in 1990, while at college. I took up an offer from the school to see a counsellor to help manage the anxiety of a first year away from home while at university. This astute counsellor (to whom I am deeply grateful) recognized that yoga might be a useful path for me in navigating the stress of college and growing into adulthood. It was indeed revelatory – a whole world opened up that I had no idea existed, and it decided the direction of my life. Through the practice of yoga, I was drawn towards a way of living and being that was completely foreign to my upbringing in a fairly small town in Texas. Before this time, I had random glimpses of this expanded reality that yoga offered me, sensed through the raw and spacious beauty of the High Plains of the Texas Panhandle and the transcendent experience when I danced; I discovered yoga was a means to access a state that felt utterly alive and connected. Simply expressed, yoga called to me.

I spent four years exploring, discovering and learning at Mills College in Oakland, California (a remarkable women's college devoted to the education and thriving of women) and graduated with top honours with a BA in Dance. It was in the non-academic time outside class that yoga insinuated its way into the fabric of my life – a constant companion in an unfolding and deeply felt experience of wholeness. I decided to dive in deep...

When I graduated, I made the decision to live and study yoga full time in a meditation ashram in upstate New York (ashram translates from Sanskrit to mean 'without fatigue' and refers to a focused environment where yoga is explored, studied and practised). I stayed for 12 years, immersed in the practices and teachings of the yoga tradition under the guidance of an extraordinary teacher, Gurumayi Chidvilasananda. Her teaching and inspiration have been instrumental in my evolution as a yoga teacher, and in living with a sense of ease, contentment and purpose.

Within the unique environment of the ashram, silence and stillness became 'golden' – fundamental for exploring and experiencing the subtlest of states and teachings. It was here that I discovered Restorative Yoga. While I initially found meditation practice difficult (and it was the main practice taught in this unique environment), Restorative Yoga somehow gave me a way into the meditative experience described by the texts of the tradition and taught by its teachers.

As I came from a dance background that was performance-based and injury prone, being able to simply lie down and rest supported by bolsters and blankets opened the door to an inner landscape of deep connectivity and healing. It offered me a space to experience 'fullness of being', which is the way I like to describe the vibrant power of present moment awareness.

Restorative Yoga has given me the ability to become still and spend time with myself exploring the very essence of my being – a unique way to celebrate the experience of being alive, awake and present to all that life offers. I find the stillness and space emphasized in Restorative Yoga very much encourages the refinement of perception necessary for diving deep into spiritual waters. And I am endlessly grateful for the years spent living in an ashram performing spiritual practices and cultivating a worldview that nurtures on both inner and outer levels.

In 2002, I left the cloistered life of the ashram for various reasons and moved to the United Kingdom. Reflecting back, while personal life circumstances required this transition, a motivating factor was curiosity. How well could what I learned in the ashram environment translate into the experience of 'everyday' life? To a certain extent, this question still energizes my practice; Restorative Yoga has played a central role in what I have come to describe as 'living the teachings'.

When I started leading trainings in London back in 2005, very few teachers had yet heard of this style of practice. Having led trainings for over 15 years, mainly at triyoga[1] in London, I found that many teachers who attended did not regularly practise Restorative Yoga, and were unfamiliar with the props which form an essential part.

However, after a weekend immersed in Restorative practice, most of the teachers would emerge with beaming faces and a wonderment and enthusiasm for a practice which allows space and time for introspection, slow movement and stillness. Often there was a recognition of tiredness, of the fatigue due to the demands of daily life and teaching. Restorative practice allows time to recognize what is present and offers a space for renewal.

I have also noticed over the years that there seems to be an absence of the essential knowledge of alignment necessary to instruct safe and comfortable

---

1   triyoga is one of the largest yoga centres in Europe and serves as a hub for the many different styles of yoga flourishing in the West. For over 20 years it has been a home to many, myself included, wishing to deepen their expression and experience of yoga.

postures. There are many factors perhaps contributing to this dearth: the prevalence of yoga trainings led by inexperienced teachers; trainings that are short (i.e. learn how to teach yoga in one month); faster flowing styles which are unable to accommodate alignment instruction; and the influence of fitness, which has created a form of 'fitness yoga' that emphasizes 'working out' versus going deeper into embodied experience. This dichotomy perhaps is not new in the evolution of yoga, but is worrisome with regard to modern trends moving further away from the original intent of the tradition.

Restorative Yoga provides the perfect conditions for discovering alignment based on the uniqueness of an individual body that is *felt* rather than seen. It creates the conditions for softness, releasing deeply held tension that contributes to restricted movement and breath patterns; it cultivates the sensitivity and acceptance needed to work with the body's natural expression, rather than against it.

For all these reasons, I would like to offer a book that may help shift the narrative with regards to the value of this style of practice and its ethos, and re-position it within the yoga community itself. The discipline of a Restorative practice can become a radical act of self-care much needed in the normal intensity of full-time yoga teaching. It can also begin to shift the culturally driven work ethic to one that values rest, space and relaxation as a source of creativity and productivity. It gives time and space for developing the acuity of the felt sense – understanding the nuance of the body's expression and its needs – highlighting the value of slow, mindful and conscious practice. And finally, this discipline attends to the deeper layers of being so much part of the richness of the tradition that when practised, can source lasting happiness.

By practising Restorative Yoga regularly, the modern yoga teacher can affirm balanced living based on direct personal experience offering practical methods for relaxation and rest. A personal commitment to Restorative practice embraces softness, slowing down and subtlety of perception, all necessary for living in a way that inspires others to choose balanced living. In essence, Restorative Yoga can provide a method for self-regulating the nervous system, and tapping into the ever-deeper layers of experience which arise through stillness and space, naturally drawing forth a sense of purpose and meaning.

While Restorative Yoga is a relatively recent development in the evolution of yoga, I don't feel it's so very far from what the 'yogis of old' were practising.

These yogis seemed to understand the importance of a mind that was clear, calm and focused – a natural expression of a balanced nervous system – as a means to experience subtler and subtler states of being.

Restorative Yoga presents a unique amalgamation of the earlier tradition and modern postural yoga – it provides a way to approach the practice not only from a physiological point of view, but from a spiritual one. The stillness and space offer a practical and direct way to re-align the body and radically shift perception through a nervous system in balance contributing to a sense of wholeness and peacefulness hinted at by the texts of the tradition.

Perhaps because of my early ashram experience of being immersed in yoga as a way of living, Restorative Yoga has become ever more important to me over the years of my *sādhana* (spiritual practice); as a method it has provided a useful framework for me to explore the subtleties of experience, breath, embodiment, balance and, ultimately, connection.

This book will be most helpful for teachers and experienced practitioners and those interested in learning more about Restorative Yoga. It's both practical and experiential. It's arranged into three parts designed to help readers understand: (I) the history, purpose, power and characteristics of the practice; (II) its feel and expression echoing the earlier tradition with an emphasis on breath, process and presence; and (III) how to structure a successful practice/class, which includes a basic curriculum from which to build sequences, as well as the art of teaching Restorative Yoga.

Parts I and II end with enquiries and exploration about how to practically apply the knowledge learned. This helps the reader to understand their own concepts or cultural imprints, as well as their own unique patterns of holding and breath which may interfere with the ability to downshift the nervous system and, ultimately, relax – all necessary preparations for being able to teach Restorative Yoga.

Much of the anatomy and physiology that is presented in this book comes from the tireless and dedicated efforts of Chris Swain, my fearless teaching partner for over a decade in the Restorative Yoga teacher trainings, and also on the triyoga teacher trainings. He has been a steady and calm presence in his indefatigable presentation of the benefits of Restorative Yoga, and I am truly grateful for his contribution to the work.

In the end, this book describes the power, presence and practice of Restorative Yoga, clarifying its expression in relation to other styles of practice. It's my hope that through this book more yoga teachers will start to practise Restorative Yoga with confidence and feel able to share its benefits with others, and that we as a collective of yoga teachers across the world can create safe spaces where students are able to come to class, slow down and experience the gift of space and stillness.

Part I

POWER

To lie down, pause, become still and feel...allows the physiology of the body to downshift into a balanced state sowing the seeds for connection, creativity and heart-felt contentment.

Chapter 1

History of Restorative Yoga

PAST AND PRESENT

Considering the present with respect to history and tradition gives a sense of why things are the way they are. It also establishes the strength of a source which informs future innovations. Within the context of yoga, the tradition provides a unity which determines whether a new style of practice links back while adapting to time, place and need, or diverges and becomes something entirely different. In my opinion, Restorative Yoga links back and honours the tradition in a fresh and new way.

While it's beyond the remit of this book to go into the full details and nuance of the history of yoga – it's a long one which gives credence to its status as a tradition – there are many great academics, historians and scholar-practitioners who have done so and continue to, research, translate and write about yoga, mapping its rich past and helping make sense of its present.[1]

This chapter touches on a few salient points in yoga's history that contextualize the emergence of Restorative Yoga. Modern postural yoga (of which Restorative Yoga is part) comes from a long, complex and varied lineage with overlapping narratives. What is practised today represents a unique 'transnational movement' as described by Mark Singleton in his seminal book, *Yoga Body: The Origins of Modern Postural Practice* (2010). His book offers an

---

1   See Alter, J. (2004) *Yoga In Modern India: The Body between Science and Philosophy*, Princeton, NJ: Princeton University Press; De Michelis, E. (2004) *A History of Modern Yoga: Patañjali and Western Esotericism,* London: Continuum; Mallinson, J. and Singleton, M. (2017) *Roots of Yoga*, London: Penguin Random House; Singleton, M. (2010) *Yoga Body: The Origins of Modern Postural Practice*, New York, NY: Oxford University Press; Sjoman, N.E. (1996) *The Yoga Tradition of Mysore Palace*, New Delhi: Abhinav Publications.

enlightening explanation of the roots of modern yoga practice which it behooves all modern yoga teachers to read.[2]

Complex socio-political and economic forces, as well cultural movements, gave rise to the 20th-century yoga masters who have left their indelible mark on modern yoga's evolution. Add to this a rapidly globalizing world under the influence of capitalism and the advent of technology, and modern yoga has flourished across boundaries remaining remarkably intact. It has become something of a global metaphor for peace or balance enfolded within a physical practice which demonstrates the strength of yoga's formidable tradition and the universality of its teachings.

Absorbing new practices alongside traditional ones, 21st-century yoga demonstrates the tradition's history of innovation, thriving in new terrain while evolving to meet the times, as can be seen in the rapid move to 'online' from 'in-person' teaching during the recent coronavirus pandemic. Restorative Yoga finds itself uniquely placed within this context to meet the challenges posed by modern living.

B.K.S. IYENGAR AND RESTORATIVE YOGA

Restorative Yoga seems to be a relatively recent development in yoga's long history. Much of its modern expression can be attributed to the seminal work of Bellur Krishnamachar Sundararaja (B.K.S.) Iyengar (1918–2014). Described by Frederick Smith and Joan White in Singleton and Goldberg's *Gurus of Modern Yoga* (2014, p.122) as 'the most visible and influential figure in the expansion of *haṭhayoga* (i.e. postural yoga) in 20th century yoga', Iyengar helped to popularize and spread yoga when he brought his style of practice to the West in the mid-1950s. He became renowned for his assiduous practice, precision and methodology in teaching the *āsanas*, as well as his skill in treating injuries and various conditions through yoga.

---

2   'Transnational' yoga is more fully explained in Mark's book. When I first read *Yoga Body*, I remember feeling disoriented as it completely shifted my understanding of where yoga came from. I had assumed the ancientness of yoga as its authority – which it is – but nothing is ever as straightforward as you'd like to think! I highly recommend reading his book in order to begin to consider and better understand the complexity of modern yoga's roots. Be sure to read his subsequent commentary in the Preface to the 2016 Serbian edition of *Yoga Body* (2015, Belgrade: Neopress Publishing) where he addresses some of the questions raised by his book.

As a young boy, Iyengar was adversely affected by the 1918 influenza pandemic. His mother caught the disease during pregnancy, which resulted in him being sickly for much of his childhood. At the age of 15 he was invited to Mysore by his brother-in-law, Tirumalai Krishnamacharya, to study yoga and improve his health through its practices.

Krishnamacharya is referred to as 'the father of modern yoga',[3] and studying yoga in Mysore under Krishnamacharya's tutelage changed the direction of Iyengar's life, setting him on a path as a major player in the evolution of 20th-century yoga. In 1937, at the age of 18, Iyengar (2005) went to Pune to 'spread the teaching of yoga' (p.xix).

Iyengar's access to Krishnmacharya's teaching during his time at Mysore and after was limited. This not only created the conditions for Iyengar to find his own interpretation and expression of yoga, it also gave rise to his innovative genius. Gradually, Iyengar unfolded his own unique style of yoga using creativity and determination to overcome the different challenges he faced. In his inspiring book, *Light on Life* (2005), he says: '...[My] body became my first instrument to know what yoga is. My own body was the laboratory... I could already see that yoga would have as many benefits for my head and heart as it did for my body' (p.xx).

Working with a diverse range of students, including those who were ill or managing medical conditions, Iyengar created 'props' to adapt the yoga practice, rendering poses more accessible, stable and easeful. He also worked extensively and imaginatively with props in his own practice to deepen his experience of *āsana* and perception in order to realize the more subtle states expounded by the texts of the tradition. His prodigious skill in both regards gave birth to Restorative Yoga, notable for its use of props, focus on nervous system health and deep interiority.

A BIT ABOUT PROPS

The primary props used in Restorative Yoga today are blankets, bolsters, belts and blocks, which are a direct result of Iyengar's creative innovation.

---

3   For an interesting article on Krishnamacharya see Mohan, A.G. (5 April, 2017) 'Memories of a master,' *Yoga Journal* [Nov 30, 2009], which is an excerpt from the book *Here Flows the River: The Life and Teachings of Krishnamacharya*. www.yogajournal.com/yoga-101/philosophy/memories-of-a-master.

Furthermore, Iyengar's legacy can be found in most studios around the world in the proliferation of props which aid practice.

While Iyengar can be considered the most influential teacher in 20th-century yoga to have incorporated props in a systematic way, the use of props has long been part of the history of yoga. Richard Rosen (2017) discusses how they aided the yogi in practice and offered the support needed to hold postures for longer periods of time. Common props from the tradition were walls, ropes and the *yoga daṇḍa* or crutch used to adjust nasal dominance by pressing the head of the staff into an armpit.

It was a simple cloth yoga strap, or what was known as the *yogapaṭṭa*, that was the most emblematic and ubiquitous. The image of a yogi strapped into a posture is widely present in statues at temples in India, and in images from the various texts describing *haṭhayoga*. In his illuminating article, 'The Ancient Yoga Strap: A Brief History of the Yogapaṭṭa', Seth Powell (2018) describes the yoga strap, which was used to fix the body in position for meditation, as 'an icon depicting spiritual prowess and transcendence over the limitations of the human body'.

Curiously, it seems Iyengar was unaware of this history. When travelling in the 1960s in France, he saw a luggage strap tying people's bags together and thought it would be a great prop to tie his legs. When he returned home to Pune, he created the practical square buckle strap (now used in Restorative Yoga) which allows a practitioner easy access into and out of a pose (Iyengar 2012).

For many modern yogis not familiar with Iyengar yoga, props may appear to be a foreign species looked at with trepidation during a fast and furious yoga practice – the interpretation of their use indicating less ability or agility (a distinctly modern twist contrasting with medieval yoga's notions of the strap indicating skill). When used in the Restorative sense, props provide a comforting and supportive means for gliding into a profoundly relaxed state of being, serving as an effective means for realizing the more elevated purpose of yoga practice itself – to know one's self or essential nature.

In trainings, I often get asked whether Restorative Yoga can be practised without props. I've come to the conclusion that it can't, because of its history and because of how the props themselves support the relaxation response and refinement of perception. There are ways to adapt a practice and make it 'prop light'. (More on this in Chapter 4, Nature of the Practice.)

GENTLY, GENTLY

'*Haṭh*', which translates to mean force or violence, has led to the translation of *hathayoga* as the 'forceful' yoga. This can be a bit confusing at first, and has caused controversy in yoga's long history, with some considering it to refer to the effort required for practice.

In his 2011 article, 'The Meaning of *hatha* in Early Hathayoga', Jason Birch elucidates the matter, explaining that the forceful aspect refers to 'forcing what normally moves down (i.e., *apāna, bindu*) and what is usually dormant (*kuṇḍalinī*) to move upwards' (p.537). In others words, the practice itself is not forceful, but rather the results of its techniques – the movement of energy upwards. Birch goes further to say that 'the word *hatha* is never used in *Hatha* texts to refer to violent means or forceful effort' (p.531), but that instead what is often used to describe the nature of practice is '*śanaiḥ śanaiḥ*', which means gradually, slowly or gently, and to proceed with caution.

Furthermore, the *Haṭhapradīpikā*, the 15th-century text in which Swātmārāma unified and systematized *hathayoga* (the name which then referred to the diverse practices of yoga described in the text and which has now become a generic term for physical practice), says: 'The corpse pose (*śavāsana*) is when one lies supine on the ground like a corpse. The corpse pose takes away fatigue and relaxes the mind' (Mallinson and Singleton 2017, p.109).

Both these aspects to me are significant and reinforce my own experience of the nature and approach of yoga practice in general, and specifically Restorative Yoga. They suggest that a deep respect is required in the approach that recognizes the inherent power residing within the human body and psyche waiting to be 'awakened' – a recognition of the power extant in every cell of the body. It also gives a clear indication of the result of yoga practice – to remove fatigue and calm the mind.

Because the postures in Restorative Yoga are supported and comfortable, and held for longer periods, they encourage a state of balance which allows for what the *Haṭhapradīpikā* describes. The practice itself is mindful, soft, slow – at times still – where present awareness and the felt sense guides the process. The addition of the props offers comfort which supports restitution, allowing for the release of multi-layered tension and freedom of breath. The impact of this on the nervous system can result in a transformational shift, facilitating a deep sense of connection which may be experienced as an awakening or raising of consciousness – a certain kind of 'liberation' that is as radical as it is profound. In this sense, Restorative Yoga offers an easeful and accessible way to experience the more subtle and profound states of being which the texts of the tradition point towards.

LIMB 3 AND A HALF!

In my Restorative teacher trainings, I often playfully describe Restorative Yoga as 'Limb 3 and a half' within the framework of *Patañjali's* Eight Limbs of Yoga, to give a sense of its role in the gradual refinement of perception and preparation for the state of *samādhi* or absorption.[4]

The physicality of the postural practice (Limb 3 – *āsana*) strengthens and prepares the body and mind for a steady focus that is inwards and present (Limb 3 and a half – Restorative). The rejuvenation of the Restorative practice allows for the softness and subtlety needed for skilful breathing (Limb 4 – *prāṇāyāma*). All preparatory for mastery of the final limbs.[5]

A PERSONAL EXPERIENCE

Early in my study of yoga, I had the opportunity to train with Kevin Gardiner, one of the senior-most Iyengar yoga teachers in New York City. I would travel the two hours down from the Catskills to New York City and back again in order to study with him. I was inspired by his clarity and insight, as well as the precision of his *āsana* instruction. Kevin's artful descriptions and language invited me into the beauty of postural practice which spoke to me as a dancer and a seeker. I am very grateful for his teaching, which continues to inspire me to this day.

Kevin cleverly used props throughout his expressive sequences; I would spend hours in a café after a class trying to remember not only the sequence, but how and why he used the props. (I still consult these notes today!) This formative time showed me that props could be an integral, enlightening and fun part of yoga practice.

As the years have passed I've gravitated towards Restorative Yoga, which combines intelligent prop usage and a considered sequence with a desire to

---

4   Sometimes I think of it like platform 9¾ in Harry Potter – the secret entryway into the more subtle states of being.

5   The order of the limbs doesn't necessarily need to be consecutive, but there is a mastery of each limb that naturally leads to the success of the next. Edwin Bryant describes it as 'consecutive interdependence' (Bryant 2009, p.289).

investigate more deeply the nature of being through embodied experience. It has helped me (and still does!) navigate the vicissitudes of a highly alert nervous system and the stress of everyday living.

JUDITH LASATER

One of the very first books I came across on Restorative Yoga in the mid-1990s was *Relax and Renew* by Judith Lasater (1995). It has become a dog-eared staple on my bookshelf. One of B.K.S Iyengar's pioneering students, Judith has greatly contributed to the unfolding of Restorative Yoga further developing this unique body of work. Perhaps more than anyone, Judith has built a structure and legacy that promotes the power of Restorative Yoga.

CONCLUSION

In my teaching of Restorative Yoga over the past 20 years, there are narratives that I'd like to correct. The first is that Restorative Yoga is for people who are poorly. While it certainly promotes healing, recovery and longevity, I would like to state emphatically that this type of practice is for *everyone*. If you have a nervous system, then Restorative Yoga is for you! Part of the practice is learning about how your nervous system works, and then taking proactive and specific steps to support balance and wellbeing.

Second, I get asked again and again the difference between Restorative and Yin. While both styles of yoga are introspective, slow and 'on the floor', they come from very different branches of the ever-evolving modern postural yoga tree. They are simply different practices. Yin very specifically came into being through the creative efforts of Paul Grilley, and has found further expression through many great contemporary Yin teachers.

Confusing the matter perhaps is an ongoing inevitable cross-pollination (very much part of the yoga tradition) as yoga teachers explore and innovate based on their experience, resources and what they see is needed for their students.

What I can say is that Restorative Yoga focuses almost entirely on nervous system health, facilitating a gradual release of tension and fullness of breath, all of which help the body and mind to relax and find equilibrium. The practice itself uses a variety of props which support relaxation, placing a great deal of emphasis on comfort.

Representing a gentle, yet powerful approach to yoga practice that reflects a long history, Restorative Yoga is fast becoming a self-empowered means for navigating choppy waters, living well in times of adversity and integrating unfolding experience in order to make sense of our ever-changing world.

Chapter 2

Purpose of Restorative Yoga

MODERN TIMES

The reality of modern living leaves marks of disembodiment, disorientation and fatigue, reflecting the complexity of our times. Technology has added a virtual dimension to the one we actually inhabit – a non-physical realm that removes all aspects of grounding, as well as the vital and tangible human cues that help a nervous system 'feel safe'. The recent pandemic has furthered the reliance on technology as an interface for connection, posing a real conundrum for a nervous system which has evolved over the millennia to survive through direct contact and interaction with others.

While technology has improved many aspects of life, it seems to have taken something vital away from the quality of our living – a certain depth and quality of fullness that comes from diving deep into embodied experience. Modern times have given rise to an inability to 'switch off', slow down and stay present, revealing a nervous system chronically out of balance.

Restorative Yoga offers a direct way to help with this conundrum of disembodiment and imbalance. Much like a 'system reboot', the practice re-establishes the ability to act with energy, clarity and ease. It can shift the nervous system out of a state of defence into a physiological state that is calm and receptive – a mode of being that illuminates and re-affirms *connection*, allowing for a different experience of reality – one that feels soft, expansive and wholesome. Within this framework, beauty reveals her ineffable presence emerging from a state of equanimity, one of the earliest definitions of yoga from the *Bhagavadgītā*.

YOGA: AN EMBODIED ENQUIRY

A premise within various yoga schools and texts describes the body as a micro-cosm of the macrocosm (Mallinson and Singleton 2017). In Olivelle's (2008) translation of the *Bṛhadāraṇyaka Upaniṣad* it says, 'It is one's self which one should see and hear, and on which one should reflect and concentrate. For by seeing and hearing one's self...one gains the knowledge of this whole world' (p.29, 2.4.5). Exploring depth of experience through body and being serves not only as a means to know one's essential self, but to enter into an abiding knowledge and understanding of the whole of life, nature, the universe and so on.

While yoga offers a direct pathway to an embodied state of knowledge, Restorative Yoga offers a particularly powerful method for adjusting physio-logical state, where perception becomes clear and spacious; deeper questions about life and meaning can be engaged with through the direct sense and feel of the layers of the body and being. The slow nature of the practice lends itself to enquiry.

In this spirit, it can be helpful to first question the cultural frameworks which have formed deeply held beliefs about work versus rest. I've heard many times from students and teachers alike that Restorative Yoga isn't 'real' yoga – or that it's basically lying over a bolster and sleeping for an hour. A specific process of asking questions can reveal deep-seated beliefs or narratives that sabotage the ability to experience deep rest. The revelation that occurs through asking questions begins to shift unconscious narratives or behaviours, opening the door to the rejuvenating effect of the practice. (More in Chapter 6, *Ātmavicāra*, which explores this type of enquiry.)

Restorative Yoga allows for another type of enquiry which I am calling 'embodied presence'. This type of enquiry accesses wisdom latent within every cell of the body and being, not just the mind, through felt sense and presence. Posing a broad question at the beginning of practice with the intent to access deeper wisdom can elicit an epiphany through the course of attending unfolding experience. Questions such as, 'What is my essential nature?' or, 'Where do I begin and end?' offer an inner scaffolding for exploring and affirming the enlivening nature of conscious embodiment. (More about this in Chapter 7, Embodied Presence.)

One of my favourite questions to contemplate comes from the great 20th-century philosopher and anthropologist Gregory Bateson, who asked a fundamental question in his book *Mind and Nature* (1979, p.8) which fuelled his life's work, 'What is the pattern that connects?' I like to pose this question at the beginning of a Restorative Yoga practice, then allow the internal and quiet inner world of my own being to speak essential truths without words – an embodied enquiry anchored in presence and space.

Restorative practice can become a revelatory process of engagement with self and being. By questioning cultural frameworks and exploring the felt sense of the body and being where essence can be touched and known, practice becomes an enlightening means for uncovering universal truths at the heart of human 'being'.

INTENTION OF THE PRACTICE

Restorative Yoga can be practised by anyone. It provides a vital support for nervous system health, allowing time for rejuvenation and connection. A powerful (and perhaps radical) act of self-care, it promotes resilience and prioritizes relaxation fundamental to wellbeing, drawing forth a state of evenness which re-affirms the time-honoured teachings of the tradition.

Over the years, I've asked teachers who've come to the Restorative teacher training to come up with an intention they might hold when planning and teaching a Restorative class, and some beautiful intentions have been shared. The following is one that has served me well over the years, helping to create classes that resonate with the power of this unique practice:

The intention in a Restorative Yoga class is to create an environment of calm, quiet and simplicity that brings about a slowing down of the nervous system through gentle, slow stretches and Restorative postures. The outcome of a practice results in a relaxed, grounded and centred state which supports nervous system health, alongside a sense of wellbeing, clarity and connection.

BROAD CHARACTERISTICS

I also ask in my trainings, 'How would you describe this practice to someone new?' This starts a dialogue which helps to shed light on the practice, as well as its effect. Teachers start by sharing a word or two which encapsulates their experience: peaceful, soothing, grounding, releases tension, spacious, nurturing and so on. So, how is Restorative Yoga different from a regular yoga class? There are some broad overarching characteristics of the practice that help distinguish it from other styles. (Chapter 4, Nature of the Practice, describes this in more depth.)

Postures are usually (but not always) 'on the ground', either supine or prone, and in this respect support a grounded and centred state. I rather like Bessel van der Kolk's definition of what it means to be grounded written in his book, *The Body Keeps the Score* (2014, p.70), '"Grounded" means that you can feel your butt in your chair, see the light coming through the window, feel the tension in your calves, and hear the wind stirring the tree outside.' I think it's helpful to think of grounding in this way – an acute sense of present moment awareness where the mind and the body are in the same place, and in contact with the earth.

The body is supported by various props which offer a sense of comfort, care and the ability to rest; poses are *always* supported in some way to ensure a safe sense of letting go where stillness and silence pervade the perceptual space. Characterized by longer holdings which give time for shifting the nervous system towards 'rest and digest', supported postures allow time to gradually release muscular tension bringing about the relaxation response so necessary for rejuvenation, balance and a sense of wellbeing.

Restorative practice presents a much slower and more introspective approach than a modern *vinyasa* practice. The primary sense perception is touch – and expansion of the felt sense – rather than sight. The eyes are closed for the majority of the practice and the trajectory of the perception is inwards towards the essence of being.

In summary, poses are generally lying down, supported by props that offer comfort and ease. Downshifting the nervous system remains at the heart of the practice, which lends itself to the search for self and meaning.

In Restorative Yoga, the general rule is 'less is more'.

THE IMPORTANCE OF SLOWING DOWN, AWARENESS AND BREATH

Restorative Yoga offers an acute sense of the present moment as it unfolds to the extent that it feels as if time slows down. The fullness of a moment reveals itself through simplicity, a sense of support and taking time. A singular focus unwraps the interrelationship between body, psyche and awareness – beyond a sense of individual identity and the forms of thoughts. Much time in Restorative Yoga is spent feeling into what is present through the lens of spacious awareness.

There is a chapter in one of the Harry Potter books when Dumbledore draws all his thoughts and memories out of his head with his wand and places them carefully into a magic bowl (remember Harry fell into it?) as a way to experience space. To me, this is the magic wand of Restorative Yoga – thoughts, ideas, memories, concepts and fears can get set aside for a short while to experience the space of a vibrant and felt 'present'.

Feeling into the texture and shape of a given moment through awareness and breath begins to shift the sense of the body from its form to its essence. The subtleties of the breath provide a softly flowing pathway inwards – a slow savouring of each moment. The interplay of an inhale and exhale reveals an underlying spaciousness that dissolves the sense of feeling separate or lacking in some manner – an inner realm compelling in its quality of fullness and completeness. This is the power of Restorative Yoga – a profound 'awakening' to life from the stance of wholeness where the outcome of the practice gifts clarity, insight and resolution.

BENEFITS OF THE PRACTICE

- Calms

- Grounds

- Centres

- Relieves stress and promotes balance

- Removes fatigue and rejuvenates

- Refreshes perception and promotes a positive outlook

- Aids sleep

- Releases tension and cultivates softness/openness

- Improves breathing and a sense of vitality

- Helps manage anxiousness and restlessness

- Supports immune system function

- Helps to shift the 'survival' or stress response towards homeostasis or balance

- Promotes the relaxation response, shifting the metabolism to 'rest and digest'

- Supports a balanced and resilient nervous system

- Increases a sense of wellbeing, joy and vibrant aliveness

- Encourages purposeful and balanced living

- Provides a means for self-enquiry that reaffirms a sense of place, purpose and meaning

- Cultivates the ability to fully experience and enjoy the moment, as well as connect with others

- Strengthens the experience of interconnection and interrelationship through embodied presence and conscious awareness.

Chapter 3

Understanding the Stress Response

INTRODUCTION

Restorative Yoga offers a method of practice that helps return the body and mind to a state of balance by encouraging the relaxation response and recruiting the body's natural physiological systems (notably the regulatory neuroendocrine systems) to support equilibrium. The concept of stress, homeostasis and the neuroendocrine system are further described in this chapter in order to shed light on how the practice of Restorative Yoga can support the movement towards balance, as well as refine its practice and teaching. It's important to recognize that the physiology of the body is highly complex and interconnected; the topics touched on in this chapter have been simplified in order to be better understood.

THE CONCEPT OF STRESS

Before starting to unwrap the workings of the stress response, it's worth taking a few minutes to consider what stress actually is and how to recognize its signs in daily life. Before reading any further, reflect on your understanding of stress and how you, and others close to you, may experience it.

There is a general consensus that stress can be recognized by the following:

- Chronic anxiety, worry and panic

- Broken sleep patterns – nocturnal anxiety waking in the early hours worrying, insomnia or sleeping too much

- Feeling overwhelmed and unable to cope – losing perspective and making 'mountains out of molehills'

- Negative outlook and catastrophic thinking

- Irritability and aggression – being critical and easily triggered

- Poor digestion and erratic eating patterns – drawn to sugar and carbohydrate snacks

- Poor judgement and concentration – being easily distracted

- Memory problems

- Uncertainty – the feeling of not being in control

- Isolating oneself from others – the feeling of not having the energy to be with people

- Procrastination and prevarication – neglecting responsibilities and not completing tasks

- Lowered immunity – vulnerability to frequent colds

- Tension headaches

- Rapid heart beat (panic attacks) and raised blood pressure

- Nervous habits – nail biting, pacing, grinding teeth and jaw clenching

- Use of alcohol, caffeine, cigarettes or drugs.

The government Labour Force Survey from March 2020 states that 17.9 million working days were lost due to work-related stress, depression or anxiety in Great Britain, with 828,000 workers being affected over 2019/20. These numbers reflect the profound effect that stress can have on health and wellbeing, and the relevance of Restorative Yoga as a practice to help manage its debilitating effects.

The etymology of the word 'stress' offers a visceral sense of its experience – it derives from the Middle English word *destresse*, which comes from the Latin word *stringere* meaning 'to draw tight' (Barnhart 1988, p.1075). 'Stress' has entered modern language with phrases like, 'I'm stressed out', 'workplace stress' and 'post-traumatic stress disorder'. Stress in and of itself is not necessarily a bad thing; in small doses it can help performance and motivation. What emerges in the conversation about stress involves a range between 'good' stress and 'bad' stress, which very much depends on individual limits and capacity. In this regard, it's important to articulate that the *experience* of stress varies widely, and depends on an individual's ability to tolerate pressure. What may be seen as a negative amount for one person, may well be seen as a positive and stimulating amount for another. However, the word 'stress' in modern times has generally become associated with the negative.

Used commonly in everyday language, stress has become increasingly difficult to define. Referred to in both biological and psychological sciences, it has become an 'umbrella term' sharing some common meaning, as well as covering a spectrum of conditions and contexts. The topic of stress is broad, complex and multifaceted; it involves complicated psycho-social and economic factors in addition to complex individual physiological and psychological makeup. One of the emerging key themes in the field of stress underlines the importance of understanding the uniqueness of individual makeup, biological constitution, history, perception and circumstances.

THE HISTORY OF STRESS

Before the 1920s, the word stress held none of its modern connotations; it was originally used in physics and engineering to refer to the internal distribution of force exerted on a material body resulting in strain. Modern stress research can be traced back to the early 20th century and the work of Hungarian endocrinologist Hans Selye (1907–1982), who first popularized and shaped the term stress (albeit with some controversy) after it had been introduced in the biological context by Walter Cannon and the early pioneering work of Claude Bernard, among others (Cantor and Ramsden 2014).

Described in his first scientific publication on adaption and disease in *Nature* in 1936, Selye conducted endocrinological experiments in Montreal, which involved injecting mice with irritating substances. He observed that the injections produced the same symptoms – swelling of the adrenal cortex, atrophy of the thymus, and gastric and duodenal ulcers – as in people when exposed to 'noxious agents', which he later coined as 'stress'.

In his article, 'The general adaptation syndrome and the diseases of adaptation' (1946), Selye describes three phases of non-specific physiological response to a noxious stimulus (stress):

- *Alarm* – when the body recognizes there is danger and prepares to deal with the threat to its survival through an instant 'fight or flight' response.

- *Resistance (Adaptation)* – when the body adapts or becomes resistant to chronic stress as a means of coping, and starts to function as if it were normal.

- *Exhaustion* – when the reserves of the body become exhausted and health starts to fail resulting in illness, which causes more stress. This can be a 'fast drop' phase with a serious breakdown in health.

Stemming from this earlier research, Selye eventually developed the concept of positive stress as 'eustress' and negative stress as 'distress' in his book *Stress Without Distress* (1974). In it he defined stress as 'the non-specific response of the body to any demand made upon it' (p.137), where illness, heat, cold, fear and injury are all equally perceived as threats.

HOMEOSTASIS

As his research on stress evolved over the years, Hans Selye acknowledged the influence of the work of Claude Bernard, who developed the idea of the *milieu interior* in 1865, and Walter Cannon's concept of homeostasis described in his book, *The Wisdom of the Body* (1932).

Homeostasis acts like a domestic thermostat stopping a house from getting too cold or too hot, serving as a regulatory system that maintains the balance of physiological systems fundamental to health. The concept of homeostasis lies at the core of the theory of the physiological mechanism of stress, which describes a stressor as something that knocks the body out of homeostatic balance. It can be physical, physiological or psychological – anything from an increase in temperature to struggling to meet mortgage repayments. The stress response is designed to re-establish homeostatic balance, a necessary response in order to survive. Restorative Yoga supports this physiological movement in regaining balance.

The concept of homeostasis came from Bernard's idea of the 'milieu internal' published in 1865 (1974, p.84) where he said, 'The constancy of the internal environment is the condition for a free and independent life.' First Bernard, and later Cannon, described the concept of homeostasis as the property of a system to regulate its internal environment and maintain stable constant conditions.

As warm-blooded mammals, humans regulate their internal physiological environment intrinsically through the autonomic nervous system (ANS) and the endocrine system in order to maintain life – these conditions necessarily include internal body temperature control around 36.8°C (called thermoregulation) and pH levels of 7.35–7.45. This ability allows human beings to have a degree of freedom to live in and adapt to a variety of external environments ranging from the extremes of the Sahara Desert to the Arctic Circle. To maintain equilibrium, multiple dynamic adjustments and regulatory mechanisms are required – an elaborate and complex sensory feedback mechanism constantly balancing the internal environment in relation to external changes. This isn't possible for cold-blooded animals, which by definition have to conform to the fluctuations of the outer environment.

Key to the regulation of the body's systems is the notion of balance. There is a certain range of physiological norms within which life can be sustained. A good example is body temperature – a human's average body temperature is 36.8°C. If body temperature goes above 44°C, death will certainly ensue, with cardio-respiratory collapse. If it goes below 26°C the heart will stop functioning. Within this range, various states of physiological dysfunction and breakdown start to occur. It is vitally important that the body applies regulatory mechanisms which keep its temperature at around 36.8°C. Mediated by the neurological and endocrinal systems, these mechanisms include sweating, shivering, panting, vasodilatation or vasoconstriction.

These regulatory physiological responses that maintain life also form the mechanisms for the stress response. Before investigating the physiological effects of the stress response, let's explore the impact of stress on performance.

THE HUMAN FUNCTION CURVE

Selye's concept of the General Adaptation Syndrome influenced a cardiologist called Dr Peter Nixon working at Charing Cross Hospital in London. He produced the Human Function Curve as a way to describe the relationship between performance and stress arousal; it offers a helpful way to conceptualize the impact of stress.

Initially, there is a positive response to stress as it enhances performance, increasing productivity coupled with the satisfaction of success and achievement. (Note that some people refer to the first section of the graph as the 'drone zone', indicating that without sufficient challenges or stimulation, there is boredom, lethargy and a lack of commitment.) The graph demonstrates that up to a point, increased stress results in increased productivity and satisfaction. However, when the level of stress starts to be greater than the ability to deal with it positively (the hump), the negative effects of stress manifest with exhaustion or 'burnout', physical/mental ill health and breakdown.

Addressing cultural attitudes towards work and rest, as well as learning how to recognize the signs of stress early, can serve society and support wellbeing. Having tools in place to help manage stress, such as a practice like Restorative Yoga, supports the body's natural physiological mechanisms, as well as the experience of living in balance.

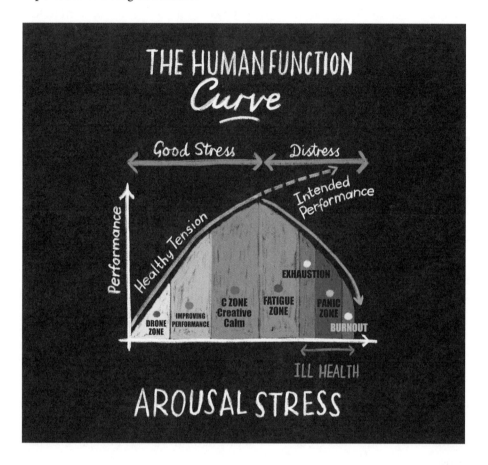

Beginning to understand the negative impact of using the term 'stress' casually can camouflage its stealthy presence. J.M. Koolhaas and colleagues (2011), in their article, 'Stress revisited: A critical evaluation of the stress concept', propose that 'the term stress should be restricted to conditions where an environmental demand exceeds the natural regulatory capacity of an organism' (quote from the Abstract) and, in this way, can clarify the use of the term.

In order to better understand the concept of stress and by definition its opposite, relaxation, let's consider some fundamental principles of human biology and physiology.

THE STRESS RESPONSE

The stress response is a term that refers to maintaining healthy homeostatic regulation of the body essential for survival. In this regard, the body manages a multitude of highly complex interactions essential for functioning within a normal range. These interactions facilitate compensatory changes supportive of physical and psychological functioning.

Helping to maintain homeostasis, the liver is responsible for metabolizing toxic substances and maintaining carbohydrate metabolism, while the kidneys are responsible for regulating blood water levels, re-absorption of substances into the blood, maintenance of sodium, ion and pH levels in the blood, and excretion of urea and other wastes.

However, it is the ANS and the endocrine system – key regulatory physiological systems often referred to as the neuroendocrine system – that act together as mechanisms for the stress response to maintain homeostasis. Before looking more closely at these systems, it is worth considering what regulates the neuroendocrine system, and this directs us to the brain.

THE TRIUNE BRAIN

The triune brain refers to a diagram that has been used in behavioural biology to illustrate how the ANS and the sympathetic nervous system (SNS) are regulated. It is a popularized oversimplification, but it helps to conceptualize what happens, especially with regard to the ANS. The first level of the triune brain includes the hypothalamus and the brain stem and regulates heart rate and respiration. It's often referred to as the 'reptilian brain'. The second layer involves the limbic system, which relates to emotions. These first two layers oversee the survival response. Finally, the third layer is the cortex, which has to do with the abstract mind – reasoning and philosophy, processing, imagination and long-term memories. The cortex is the most recently evolved part of the nervous system and is highly developed in primates.

It is this capacity for abstract thought that helps to explain the complexity of stress within a modern cultural context; the same level of stress response can be triggered by a traffic jam, having financial worries, listening to music or watching a horror film, none of which involves a direct and immediate threat to survival. When stress becomes habituated over a long period of time, it's referred to as chronic, and it's this aspect which can lead to ongoing health problems.

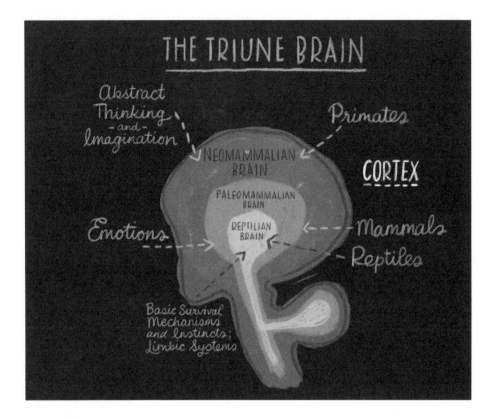

THE AMYGDALA

As a species and as individuals, human beings are fundamentally programmed to survive. The amygdala is part of the 'reptilian' or 'primitive' brain and serves as a basic survival tool; it triggers the immediate in-built survival behaviours via the hypothalamus–pituitary–adrenal axis (HPA axis), which involves 'fight or flight', and is associated with aggression, anger and fear. This is also referred to as the endocrine axis and is the hormonal response which occurs in conjunction with the SNS.

In an acute emergency situation, the stress response is essential for survival. A classic story in yogic philosophy involves mistaking a stick for a snake. When activated by fear, the amygdala overrides reasoning and initiates an immediate stress response – jump out of the way of the snake. Whether it's a snake or a rope, the same physiological response occurs prioritizing survival. The pre-frontal cortex meanwhile processes information by involving memory and learning, which it passes on to the amygdala via the thalamus; it involves a slower process. Eventually, the brain identifies that it's a rope, and shifts the physiology back towards balance.

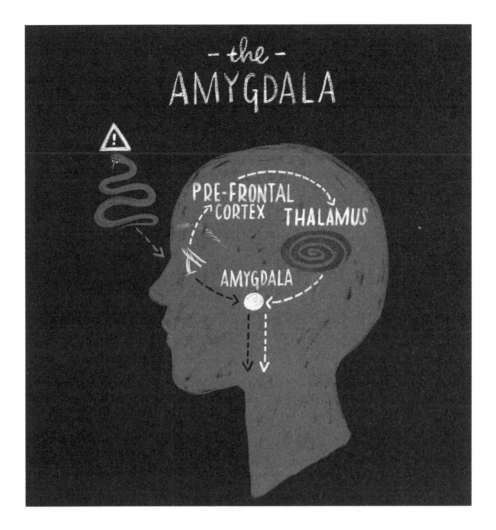

Intrinsic mental and emotional programming interweaves with survival, where the capacity for imagination and abstraction can amplify the modern-day stress response. Imagined fears, worries and insecurities switch on physiological stress mechanisms that cost a lot in terms of energy; the perception of threat through abstract and sophisticated thinking initiates the same primitive survival responses as a real physical threat. When the stress response is turned on for too long and too often, health and wellbeing deteriorate. Survival responses maintained over time result in exhaustion and breakdown; the body is not designed to be on 'red alert' over a length of time.

It's interesting to know that research by Davidson and colleagues (2008) found that Buddhist meditators who practise compassion meditation show the ability to modulate their amygdala, as shown on magnetic resonance imaging (MRI) scans. Yoga has a long history of supporting the physiology, where balance facilitates enlightened living.

THE AUTONOMIC NERVOUS SYSTEM

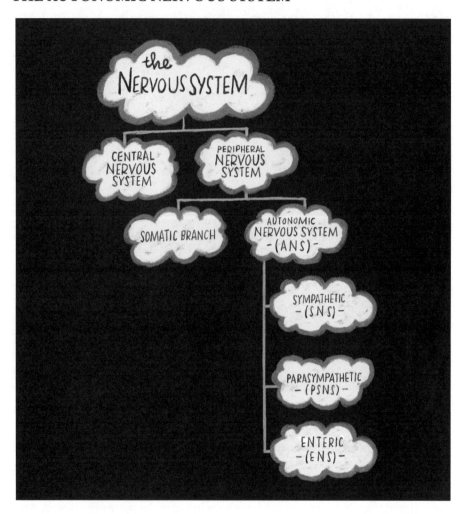

The nervous system provides the infrastructure for all sorts of self-regulation related to homeostasis using bi-directional feedback systems. The ANS ties in many biological systems and processes. For example, the ANS also includes the enteric nervous system (ENS), which is a feedback system from the gut that communicates with both neural and hormonal pathways for adjusting the physiology.

The ANS and the endocrine (hormone) system act as the key regulatory physiological systems that help to maintain homeostasis. The neuroendocrine system controls the body's internal organs. It innervates smooth muscle, cardiac muscle and glands, controlling the circulation of blood, the activity of the gastrointestinal tract, respiration, body temperature and a number of other functions. Most of this control is not conscious.

The neurological aspect of the ANS is divided into two parts, the SNS and the parasympathetic nervous system (PSNS), whose actions are mostly antagonistic. Sympathetic stimulation prepares one for survival tactics like fighting or running, commonly referred to as the 'fight or flight' response. There is also a 'freeze' response characterized by an inability to act at all; one is literally frozen, neither running away nor fighting to take action.

The nerves comprising the SNS exit the spine between T1 and L2 (T1 referring to the top thoracic vertebra of which there are 12, and L2 referring to the second lumbar vertebra of which there are five), forming a 'sympathetic chain' of ganglia. Each ganglion is like a telephone exchange centre where complex interconnected synapses occur.

The nerves forming the PSNS exit from extreme poles of the nervous system and their primary function is 'rest and digest'. There are four cranial nerves whose centres lie within the brain, and three sacral nerves exiting the sacrum at S2–4, all of which contribute to parasympathetic activity. The three sacral PSNS nerves supply the lower third of the colon, the kidneys, the bladder and the sex organs.

The four cranial PSNS nerves are:

- CN III: The oculomotor nerve – eye movement.

- CN VII: The facial nerve – facial movement.

- CN IX: The glossopharyngeal nerve – movement of the tongue and in the pharynx.

- CN X: The vagus nerve – an extensive connection to and influence over most of the major organs, including the heart, lungs, stomach, spleen and upper part of the digestive tract.

Restorative Yoga focuses on supporting the shift of the physiology from a sympathetic to a parasympathetic response. From the above innervation of the PSNS, it becomes clear how important facial expression and voice modulation are with regard to parasympathetic activity, especially in terms of teaching – an angry voice and harsh expression would be perceived as a threat and move the physiology towards an SNS response.

– AUTONOMIC NERVOUS SYSTEM –

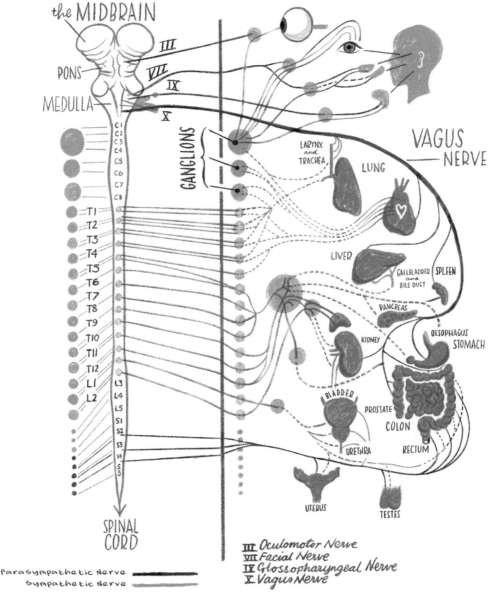

Parasympathetic Nerve ——————
Sympathetic Nerve ——————

III Oculomotor Nerve
VII Facial Nerve
IX Glossopharyngeal Nerve
X Vagus Nerve

DASHED LINE: Postganglionic Motor Neurons

SOLID LINE: Postganglionic Motor Neurons

THE ENTERIC (INTRINSIC) NERVOUS SYSTEM (ENS)

The ENS, often also referred to as the 'second brain' is one of the main divisions of the nervous system and consists of a mesh-like system of neurons that governs the function of the gastrointestinal system. While it can operate independently of the brain and the spinal cord, it normally communicates with the central nervous system (CNS) via the PSNS (e.g. the vagus nerve) and the SNS (e.g. via the pre-vertebral ganglia). Li and Owyang's (2003) research has shown that the system is operable with a severed vagus nerve.

The ENS orchestrates various gastrointestinal functions, including digestion, motility, secretion, permeability, immune and nociception (subjective perception of pain). The vast numbers of neurons in the plexi (some 500 million neurons embedded in the oesophagus and extending down to the anus) constitute the ENS, which as well as carrying out many digestive reflexes, independently mediates the influence of the brain on digestive functions and is an important part of the 'gut–brain' axis.

The gut–brain axis is a bi-directional neurohormonal communication system important in maintaining homeostasis, and is regulated through the central and enteric nervous systems and the neural, endocrine, immune and metabolic pathways, including the HPA axis. It also includes the role of gut flora as part of the 'microbiome–gut–brain axis'.

Essentially, the brain and the gut can upset each other and stress signals from the brain can alter nerve function in the gut being associated with conditions like irritable bowel syndrome (IBS), inflammatory bowel disease (IBD), heartburn and colitis. The PSNS's regulatory role, mainly carried out by the vagus nerve, seems to be primary. Its motor fibres increase intestinal activity (secretion and motility). In response to fear, the vagus will turn up the volume on serotonin circuits in the gut, and if they are overstimulated, this can result in diarrhoea. Stimulation of the pressure receptors in the gut lining results in the release of serotonin and the reflex motion of peristalsis (movement of the gut). Since 80 per cent of the activity of the vagus nerve is sensory (afferent), its numerous sensory fibres inform the brain about the condition of the gut and its content impacting the physiology.

The SNS has an inhibitory effect on the digestive system caused indirectly by constricting blood vessels in the digestive tract. The reduction in blood flow diminishes secretory and contractile activity. Both chronic stress and early life adversity can influence the microbiome–gut–brain axis.

AUTONOMIC NERVOUS SYSTEM EFFECTS
Sympathetic

- Pupils dilate

- Rate and force of heart muscle contraction increases

- Respiratory rate increased

- Lung bronchi dilate

- Metabolism increases

- Adrenal medullary secretion of adrenalin and noradrenalin increases

- Liver releases glucose

- Sweating increases

- Stomach produces fewer digestive enzymes

- Peristalsis in the gut decreases

- Digestive blood vessels constrict

- Blood shunted to peripheral muscles for action.

Parasympathetic

- Pupils constrict

- Rate and force of heart muscle contraction decreases

- Trachea and bronchial tubes constrict

- Adrenal medulla doesn't secrete

- Liver stores glucose as glycogen

- No sweating

- Metabolism is normal

- Pancreas secretes insulin and enzymes associated with gastric activity

- Secretion from salivary glands increases

- Peristalsis in the gut increases.

THE FIGHT OR FLIGHT RESPONSE

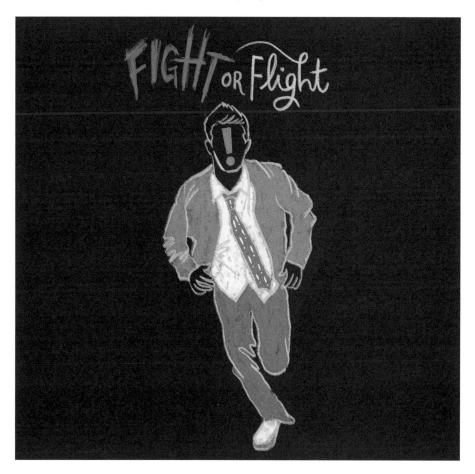

Central to the neurological component of the stress response is the SNS, which mobilizes the body's resources under stress as the fight or flight response, a fundamental part of our survival mechanism. Sympathetic stimulation is activated by any stressor that is perceived as threatening and prepares the body for emergencies like fighting or running.

The SNS helps to control most of the body's internal organs functioning beyond conscious control, regulating the fundamental processes of life like digestion and respiration. It is balanced by the PSNS, which, like a parachute, generally slows things down in the body being associated with rest and recuperation, promoting maintenance and repair. Thus, the actions of the SNS and PSNS are mostly antagonistic – for example, the SNS increases heart rate and the PSNS slows it down. These same mechanisms are essential for the regulation of homeostasis and fundamental to our survival. Restorative Yoga directly stimulates the PSNS.

THE ENDOCRINE SYSTEM

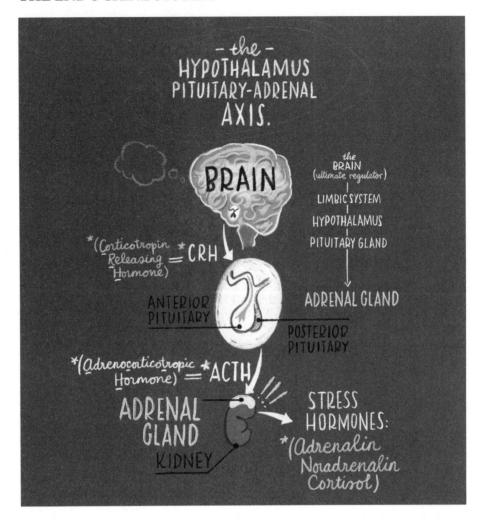

The endocrine system is responsible for the hormonal response to fight or flight. The hypothalamus, which sits just above the pituitary gland, releases corticotropin releasing hormone (CRH). This is sent to the anterior pituitary gland, which responds by releasing adrenocorticotropic hormone (ACTH), which stimulates the secretion of adrenalin, noradrenalin and corticosteroids, including cortisol, from the adrenal glands. The adrenal glands are situated on top of both of the kidneys. Hormones are blood-borne chemical messengers and affect the whole body. The following is a simplified summary of some of the effects of the stress hormones which are part of the SNS response.

- *Adrenalin* – increases heart activity, causes pupil and bronchiole dilation, vasodilation in muscles, glycogenolysis in the liver, blood clotting, vasoconstriction in the gut, kidneys, skin and so on, brain arousal and sweating.

- *Noradrenalin* – decreases digestive activity, glycogenolysis, increased heart activity, brain arousal, hair erection, rise in blood pressure, vasoconstriction in the skin, kidney, gut and so on.

- *Cortisol* – a steroid hormone (or glucocorticoid) whose primary function is to increase blood sugar through gluconeogenesis, suppress the immune system and aid in fat, protein and carbohydrate metabolism. It is also an anti-inflammatory compound inhibiting the inflammatory response, and decreases bone formation. It further enhances the effects of adrenalin in response to stress.

In an emergency situation, the overall effect of these hormones and the SNS response provides the body with physiological resources to best help survival. They increase glucose and oxygen to provide energy, and divert blood to the essential organs of the heart and brain, as well as peripheral muscles, ensuring that only those parts of the body that really need energy get it. Blood supply to the gut and other organs is reduced, as it's not central to survival. The raised blood pressure and heart rate further enhance the supply of energy.

THE VAGUS NERVE

Let's look more closely at the vagus nerve, which is the primary component of the PSNS. Known as the 'wandering nerve' (as in vagrant, a wanderer), the vagus nerve is the longest nerve of the ANS in the body. It is the tenth cranial nerve or CN X, and interfaces with the parasympathetic control of the heart, lungs, digestive organs and the upper part of the digestive tract. The first recorded mention of the vagus nerve came from Claudius Galen (130–200 AD), who lived during the time of the Roman Empire. He studied the vagus nerve as he treated gladiators, noting certain dysfunctions that occurred when it had been severed.

Pathway of the vagus nerve

On leaving the brain stem, the vagus nerve 'wanders' through the neck and chest to the gut. While there are left and right branches of the vagus nerve, they are normally referred to in the singular as the vagus nerve. Besides giving some output to various organs, the vagus nerve comprises between 80 and 90 per cent of afferent nerves mostly conveying sensory information about the state of the body's organs to the central nervous system. (Afferent nerves convey information from the body to the brain and are also referred to as 'sensory nerves'. The opposite is the efferent or 'motor nervous' system, which conveys nerve signals from the brain to the body, as in the case of the voluntary contraction of a muscle.)

Function of the vagus nerve

The vagus nerve supplies motor parasympathetic fibres to all the organs (except the adrenal glands), from the neck down to the second segment of the transverse colon (the outflow from S2–S4 supplies the lower third of the colon, the bladder and the sex organs). The vagus also controls a few skeletal muscles in the mouth and throat area. This means that the vagus nerve is responsible for such varied tasks as heart rate, gastrointestinal peristalsis, sweating and quite a few muscle movements in the mouth, including speech (via the recurrent laryngeal nerve). It also has some afferent fibres that innervate the inner (canal) portion of the outer ear (via the auricular branch, also known as Alderman's nerve) and part of the meninges.

Parasympathetic innervation of the heart is partially controlled by the vagus nerve and is shared by the thoracic ganglia. Vagal and spinal ganglionic nerves mediate the lowering of the heart rate. In healthy people, parasympathetic tone from these sources is well matched to sympathetic tone. Hyper-stimulation of parasympathetic influence promotes bradyarrhythmias – a slow resting heart rate.

Efferent vagus nerve fibres innervating the pharynx and back of the throat are responsible for the gag reflex. In addition, afferent vagus stimulation in the gut due to gastroenteritis is a cause of vomiting. The vagus nerve also plays a role in satiation following food consumption. Knocking out vagal nerve receptors has been shown to cause hyperphagia (greatly increased food intake).

Vagal tone

Vagal tone refers to the activity of the vagus nerve, specifically the continual nature of baseline PSNS action that the vagus nerve exerts. While the baseline vagal input is constant, the degree of stimulation it exerts is regulated by the baseline of inputs from the SNS and PSNS. Vagal tone is frequently used to assess heart function and is also useful in assessing emotional regulation and other processes that alter, or are altered by changes in PSNS activity. Measurements of vagal tone can be made by using the non-invasive procedure of heart rate and heart rate variability (HRV).

Heart rate variability (HRV)

It is possible to monitor vagal activity by quantifying specific rhythmic changes in the beat-to-beat heart rate pattern. HRV measures the specific changes in time (or variability) between successive heart beats. Generally, a low HRV indicates that the body is under stress from exercise, psychological events, or other internal or external stressors. Higher HRV (or greater variability between heart beats) usually means that the body has a strong ability to tolerate stress or is strongly recovering from accumulated stress. At rest, a high HRV is generally favourable and a low HRV is unfavourable. When in an active state, lower relative HRV is generally favourable, while a high HRV can be unfavourable. HRV also links cardiovascular activity to the respiratory system, digestive system, and other recovery and stress-related systems.

Polyvagal Theory

The Polyvagal Theory (PVT) was developed in 1994 by Dr Stephen Porges, Director of the Body-Brain Center at the University of Chicago. In his book, *The Polyvagal Theory* (2011), Porges describes three stages of development of the ANS, each with three major adaptive behavioural survival strategies in response to a perceived threat (stressor). Central to the theory is the observation that rather than being just one nerve, the vagus has two distinct and separate branches, which originate in two different locations, these being the 'ventral' vagus and the 'dorsal' vagus. In a model of evolutionary heritage, the three adaptive strategies describe the ANS shifting to three distinct responses which together help to maintain homeostasis.

The oldest response of the ANS involves recruitment of the dorsal vagus nerve with its slow conducting unmyelinated nerve fibres. This consists of immobilization or shutting down and would correspond to the freeze response that is seen in animals when playing dead, used as a survival mechanism. This primitive response aims to maintain metabolic resources. Immobilization with fear occurring through the dorsal vagus nerve can also be a response to trauma.

The second evolution of the ANS refers to the development of the SNS and the fight or flight response.

The most recent evolution of the ANS has to do with the neurovagal circuit and involves the 'faster' myelinated fibres of the ventral vagus nerve found only in mammals and which relate to facial expression, voice and social engagement. Perceptions of safety and/or threat are reflected in facial expression and vocal intonation. This development of the ANS allows cooperation with others, improving the chances of survival. Social engagement emphasizes making safe connections. Better living occurs when features of safety and social engagement are present, encouraging curiosity and connection rather than their opposite – strategies of shutting down, anxiety or aggression in response to perceived threats and fear. Immobilization without fear involves the ventral vagus nerve where a sense of feeling safe allows relaxation, intimacy and connection.

BARORECEPTORS AND THE BAROREFLEX

The baroreflex is one of the body's homeostatic mechanisms that helps to maintain blood pressure at nearly constant levels, providing a rapid negative feedback loop in which elevated blood pressure reflexively causes the heart rate to decrease and blood pressure to decrease. Baroreceptors are stretch-sensitive mechanoreceptors chiefly in the carotid sinus and aortic arch. Carotid sinus axons travel along the glossopharyngeal nerve (CN IX). The aortic arch baroreceptor axons travel along the vagus nerve (CN X). They both relay information to the medulla oblongata in the brain stem, and induce change in blood pressure mediated by both the SNS and PSNS.

Restorative Yoga postures recruit the baroreflex to switch to 'relaxation mode' by positioning the body in such a way that the heart is either fully or partially elevated above the head, and the neck is flexed, which initially increases blood pressure. (The vertical distance either above or below the heart determines the influence of gravity on blood pressure.) As the baroreflex registers the change, it lowers blood pressure, initiating a calming and quietening effect on the brain. To a certain extent, all supine/prone postures stimulate the baroreflex to varying degrees, depending on the angle.

THE RELAXATION RESPONSE

Dr Herbert Benson, a Harvard physician, wrote *The Relaxation Response* in 1975 with Miriam Z. Klipper and coined the phrase 'the relaxation response', the goal being to activate the PSNS, which causes humans to relax. His studies were originally prompted by Maharishi Mahesh Yogi and his students interested in researching the effects of Transcendental Meditation™.

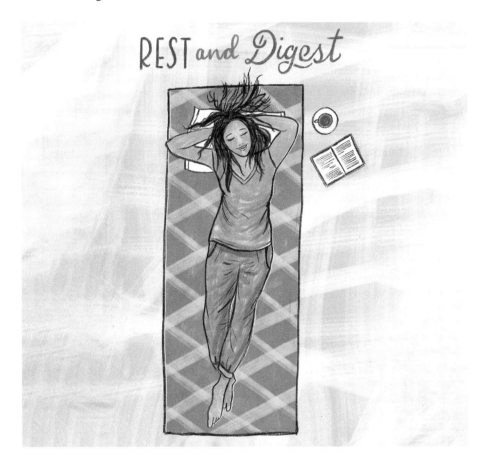

Studies by Benson showed that meditation lowered metabolic rate and blood pressure. He describes four essential components to bring about the response: a mental device (a simple word, phrase or activity to repeat to keep the mind from wandering), a passive attitude, a quiet environment and a comfortable position, the first two being essential. These 'devices' could be considered as intrinsic components of Restorative Yoga practice that shift the physiology into the relaxed state induced by the PSNS.

The ability for the mechanisms of the PSNS to balance the function of the ANS and maintain homeostasis is central to the relaxation response. If the SNS can be summarized as the 'fight or flight' response, the PSNS response can be summarized as 'rest and digest', 'tend and befriend', 'feed and breed' or 'relaxation response'.

CONCLUSION

Understanding stress and the body's response opens up a world of possibilities for how to navigate its challenges. Key in its management is understanding the individual nature of the response to stress – where one person might thrive, another might experience the same situation as incredibly stressful. Restorative Yoga can offer a powerful pathway for supporting the physiology and embracing the movement towards balance that can help reduce stress and support wellbeing.

Chapter 4

—————

Nature of the Practice

VALUING REST AND RELAXATION

The Restorative body of work facilitates wellbeing – a state of healthiness, happiness and feeling secure – where an expansive state of being allows for creativity and connection. The practice offers insight into how our nervous system works and how prolonged stress impacts health and worldviews. Stephen Porges (2020), the creator of the hugely influential Polyvagal Theory says, 'When you shift physiological state, you shift your bias of how you see the world.' Yoga teachers are well positioned to support people in understanding their own unique stress patterns, and in learning a way of practising that strengthens balance, resilience and positivity.

The nature of Restorative Yoga adeptly addresses the challenges of 21st-century living, offering ways to manage stress and highlighting the importance of rest and relaxation for living well. At the same time, Restorative practice confronts strong unconscious narratives that may sabotage the ability to relax.

The main one is that to become still and rest is somehow 'lazy'. Choosing Restorative practice is somehow 'cheating' or 'slacking off' and certainly not 'real' yoga. There may even be a belief that there isn't time to stop and rest. Or, the thought may arise, 'I'm not doing enough', equating the amount accomplished with self-worth. I have also seen students tap into a wider existential fear when they become still, provoking a certain kind of panic that disallows an open questioning about self, place, purpose and longevity.

I think it's helpful in the conversation about balance to acknowledge the complexity – where unseen cultural imprints, histories, individual capacity and survival dynamics all influence the relationship to rest and the ability to appreciate stillness. Part of the nature of the practice allows space for sitting with and questioning views with regard to a balanced life.

Taking time to become still and rest becomes a 'high-leverage' act in a culture which often devalues it. By recognizing the mental and physical impact of being 'on the go' all the time and how stress contributes to ill health and unhappiness, it's possible to shift the paradigm to one of presence and balance. Restorative practice begins to disassemble the modern work culture that covertly values 'burning the midnight oil', emphasizing getting things done over the state of connection.

More and more value is being placed on quality rest and relaxation. Restorative Yoga has begun to weave its way into the tapestry of modern living. The boom in mainstream circles of mindfulness-based stress reduction has become part of corporate and political work culture; yoga itself has become widely known for its ability to help 'de-stress', a distinctly modern interpretation of the goal of yoga – all signs of progress in dismantling a way of living that results in illness and disconnection.

While Restorative Yoga can be challenging because of our cultural norms, the stillness of the practice can bring into relief a restless or anxious mind acclimatized to stress – and this can be uncomfortable. There are those for whom becoming still and resting can be so confrontational that a faster paced style of yoga practice is necessary. The slow, introspective nature of the practice can be too much or it is simply not the right practice based on individual needs and circumstances.

While Restorative practice is exactly the type of work needed for a nervous system needing to downshift, sometimes it may be better placed *after* the more physical part of a class which helps to attenuate restlessness and tenacious thinking. This allows time to release caught energy and gradually settle into the state of stillness, which at first may seem alien and devoid of experience.

Other narratives I've heard describe Restorative Yoga as lying down and having 'a nice snooze'. This always makes me simultaneously chuckle and despair. In some ways, Restorative practice is more demanding than an active practice – students are asked to carefully re-create an unusual set-up of props, place themselves with awareness, and take into consideration the uniqueness of their own body and patterns of holding. One could argue the ability to feel subtlety, adjust and soften into an internal and felt (as opposed to seen) world is advanced work.

For some, the precision, stillness and introspection of Restorative Yoga put it on par with the challenge of meditation. A more active postural practice can provide a useful preparation for the introspection and interiority of Restorative

Yoga (remember Limb 3 and a half?). Restorative practice can cultivate a sustained inner absorption required for meditation. As with anything, it's a matter of understanding individual needs, managing expectations and at times embracing an initial discomfort that eventually dissolves with consistent practice.

Sometimes people simply fall asleep when they practise Restorative Yoga. This reveals either a deep fatigue or an inability to stay present, both of which rob the practice of its depth. And yet sleep may be what's needed and in this way Restorative practice gives what's needed. But, falling asleep during a practice can also be disturbing to both the sleeper and others in the space when the sonorous sound of a snore disturbs the collective sanctuary! There are ways to address this graciously and we will look at this in Chapter 15, The Art of Teaching Restorative Yoga.

Managing the uniqueness of an individual stress response has much to do with the nature of the Restorative work. Giving time and space to reflect on and investigate sensations, tendencies or patterns that contribute to stress is very much a part of the practice. Beginning to challenge narratives and habitual patterns that interfere with the ability to relax and go deeper allows for a new relationship with space, time, stillness and self. In this sense, Restorative Yoga addresses both perception and attitudes towards rest, as well as physiological state.

STILLNESS, QUIETUDE AND NON-DOING

The maxim 'less is more' underpins the ethos of Restorative practice. I find myself coming back to this essential truth time and again when crafting a Restorative experience where stillness and non-doing elucidate what is meant by space.

Space manifests in various ways in a Restorative class: fewer postures, quietude, breath awareness, the release of physical and mental tension, and non-doing – or rather the joy of *being*. In this regard, the pace of a class or practice is unhurried, spacious and savoured. Learning to *savour* space enlivens practice and can bring forth an inner experience of contentment that arises when 'doing' stops and 'being' takes over. This necessarily involves a paradigm shift where stillness, rather than movement, becomes the focus. One of the best ways I have found to understand and make this shift involves the breath, which expresses both aspects. It's here where deep rejuvenation, as well as joy, can be sourced. (More on this in Part II, Presence.)

In crafting a practice, I *always* consider the arrangement of the space and how to promote relaxation. I remember once visiting a Japanese spa in Northern

California; everything in the outer environment was designed to create a direct and tangible feeling of spacious presence. The simplicity and beauty of the outer environment struck me as such a powerful way to shift gears into a mode of being *receptive* to these aspects. In a Restorative class, every part of the experience is considered from the point of view of space and the nervous system – an outer spaciousness supports an inner spaciousness.

The physical environment of a Restorative class offers a direct and tangible feeling of space and offers a safe haven for rest and rejuvenation that at its essence is nourishing. Everything in the outer environment of a class, including the manner of the teacher, lends itself to calm presence. (More on this in Chapter 15, The Art of Teaching Restorative Yoga.)

In the spirit of a whole-body enquiry, it's helpful to encourage students to consider their personal experience of space and what this actually means to them. Asking the question 'What does it feel like to experience space?' can be a transformative agent in the evolution of a mindset that embraces rest as part of balanced living.

SUPPORTING THE EXPERIENCE OF RELAXATION

Considering the following aspects when practising and teaching Restorative Yoga supports a relaxed, grounded and centred state which reinforces a healthy nervous system, alongside a sense of wellbeing and connection.

Feel and follow the breath

Breath *awareness* provides the underpinning for Restorative practice, where a free and easeful breath serves as a means to turn inwards, settle and experience fullness of being. Breathing with ease sends the right kind of cues to the brain that downregulate the nervous system (especially with the focus on an exhale), supporting a sense of space and wellbeing.

Complex *prāṇāyāma* techniques may actually cause stress. 'Controlling' the breath or even trying to 'breathe properly' often results in grasping for it, which interferes with the breath's natural movement and rejuvenating power. There is no need to 'do' the breath; there is no need to control or force the breath. Rather, follow the natural expression of the breath and lightly accent what is already happening, reaffirming the innate intelligence of the breathing body.

As the cornerstone of Restorative practice, the breath gives the mind an all-important focus during practice other than its thoughts and worries. When felt and followed, the breath becomes a pathway into a state of connection. Bessel van der Kolk, in his book *The Body Keeps the Score* (2014), describes the power of present moment awareness combined with the felt sense as a way to powerfully adjust physiological state. Following the breath's texture and flow allows this combination, which helps focus, calm and quiet the mind.

Both the inhale and the exhale are 'hardwired' to the nervous system – the inhale slightly activating, the exhale calming. Striking the balance between these two expressions of the breath cultivates evenness and calm presence. Gently lengthening the exhale without forcing supports calming; lingering at the end of an exhale can deepen the relaxation response.

Sometimes, there may be a breathing pattern disorder that interferes with the fullness of the breath's expression. This can happen through illness, trauma or prolonged stress. Skipping the all-important practice of breath awareness can further embed an underlying breathing pattern disorder and cause greater disturbance to the nervous system. An approach that explores the experience of breathing without judgement, and that encourages what is natural, may be revelatory and shift an anxious or disturbed breath pattern.

When possible, breath through the nose on both the inhale and exhale. The crisp coolness of the inhale and soft warmth of the exhale works very well as a focus during practice. Nose breathing filters, warms and humidifies the breath preparing it for the lungs. It creates a soft resistance that slows and naturally amplifies the breath. Interestingly, it's also where nitric oxide, a vasodilator, gets produced, which supports oxygen transport and the widening of smooth muscles and blood vessels, all helpful for relaxation.[1]

To support more efficient breathing and the ability to rest, focus on the pulsation of the diaphragm encouraging a quieting of the shoulders, neck and face. The diaphragm is sometimes referred to as the second heart, and its movement centres the mind within the feel of the body and supports calming. Placing the hands on the solar plexus brings awareness to patterns of holding that may

1   Over the years, I have found the online website SequenceWiz, created by Olga Kabel, an amazing resource for learning and applying that learning to teaching yoga. I highly recommend signing up for her newsletter. Olga's dedication, knowledge and insight are incredibly clear and supportive, and I am grateful to her ongoing contribution and efforts. Kabel, O. (8 July, 2020) Nose vs mouth breathing: Which one is better for your Health? Yoga for Your Energy, Sequence Wiz, https://sequencewiz.org/2020/07/08/nose-vs-mouth-breathing-which-one-is-better-for-your-health.

interfere with the diaphragm's free movement; the external sense of the breath's movement through the hands adds depth and dimension to the experience.

The breath is never forced in Restorative Yoga, but felt and followed. A free and easeful breath cradles and comforts the mind, promoting evenness and relaxation. (More on breath in Part II, Presence.)

Release unnecessary tension

Mindful, slow stretches combined with breath awareness help break tensional patterns of ingrained response, providing an effective way to shift out of an overstimulated and fearful state. Chronic tension sends the message to the brain that the body should be ready to respond to a perceived threat. This type of response hardens the body and pulls it away from the ground, its source of stability. It takes a tremendous amount of energy to maintain this type of stance, which further reinforces patterns of holding and unnecessary tension.

Encourage 'the power of yield', a conscious release into gravity which promotes softness, openness and agency. To be able to move with gravity releases the resistance that costs so much in terms of energy and focus; patterns of holding can give way to softness and a visceral sense of grounding, transforming self-limiting narratives written in the tissues of the body. The inherent power of yield becomes a rejuvenating and amplifying force of connection and expansion.[2]

There are a number of key places in the body that commonly hold tension – shoulders, neck, hands, face, eyes, tongue, solar plexus and pelvic floor to name a few. Restorative practice allows time to explore, make known and release unique patterns of holding that contribute to chronic stress.

Slow stretches placed at the beginning of a sequence can help release unconscious tension and encourage depth of experience. Instruction and adjustments throughout the practice encourage further release, which supports a free and easeful breath and the ability to relax. This contributes to an emerging sense of integration and a directly felt sense of space and freedom. (More on this in Chapter 10, A Free and Easeful Breath.)

---

2   I am extremely grateful to the wonderful Jean Hall, a brilliant yoga teacher, my friend and teaching partner. Her influence on my teaching in our collaborations over the years has taught me the importance of the 'power of yield'.

Choose comfort

Comfort serves as a guiding principle in practice and as the foundation for relaxation. Understanding the Restorative set-up and the 'right' way to adjust the body to suit individual needs creates the conditions for softening, turning inwards and entering into spacious presence. Adjusting the body for comfort quiets the mind, encouraging subtlety of perception. It symbolizes a self-nurturing and empowered act – a conscious choice and movement towards balance.

Adapting the set-up of a Restorative posture forms a large part of the skill in practice and teaching. If there is a 'niggle' in any part, the mind will be pulled towards discomfort and the ability to remain settled in a pose will disappear. There is always a way to adapt, shift or change a pose in order to feel comfortable and relax.

Sometimes a liberating kind of 'discomfort' can arise even when the body is comfortable – where embedded emotions from past experience rise to the surface in the space of stillness. The question of whether to stay or come out when this type of discomfort arises boils down to physiological state. If resting in a posture results in disturbance, and adjustments or modifications do not help, then it's best to come out and change the posture entirely or take a break from the practice. There's no point in remaining in a pose or wider practice when the nervous system goes on the defensive – it defeats the wider purpose of Restorative practice. In the end, this sage advice from *Patañjali* can offer clarity, 'Posture should be steady and comfortable' (Bryant 2009, p.283, II.46).

Ground and support the body

Stabilizing and supporting the structure can create a cocoon-like effect which allows for deep rest and healing. By using various props to ground and support, the body can soften and 'let go', reinforcing feelings of comfort and safety which profoundly affect physiology. The tactile sense of being held allows for feelings of nurture and trust that can envelope the whole body and being.

A grounding prop can gently move the skeletal structure towards a more comfortable position, where muscles release their grip on the bones. In addition, a weighted prop placed on the body can restore a sense of the body itself, where the movement of the breath can be felt, experienced and savoured.

Grounding the body moves it into closer connection with the earth. 'Earthing' the body literally draws forth the settled and weighted aspect of this element, where the body, rather than being pulled down by gravity, feels its support.

Acting in much the same way as a 'gravity' blanket, weight strategically placed on the body through sandbags, bolsters or folded blankets, grounds and swaddles, helping to release chronic tension (Ackerley, Badre and Olausson 2015).

Supporting the body is an aspect of grounding. Any part of the body that is hanging against gravity will eventually tire and tense, pulling the mind out of relaxation and the body into discomfort. Actively using props such as rolled towels, folded or 'scrunched' blankets, or buckwheat bolsters lends structural support that allows the body to soften, making it possible to stay in a pose.

Placing a light weight on the eyes or brow has a quieting effect on the thinking mind. It releases unconscious facial tension, which supports the relaxation response. Light downward pressure in this area relaxes the forehead and eyes, quieting the pre-frontal cortex, that part of the brain which plans, creates and problem solves. The calming effect of this type of prop helps turn the focus inwards and away from outer objects to an internal felt sense which helps regulate state. Note: avoid placing weight directly on the eyes if there are lenses or astigmatism.

A lightness of body and being arises from the experience of being grounded and supported. Careful prop choice and placement helps free the grip of muscles and mind necessary for rest and restitution. (See Chapter 13, The Six Main Restorative *Āsana* and Variations, for more specific adjustments on grounding and supporting.)

Create a sanctuary for practice

It's essential from the point of view of the nervous system to create an environment that supports feeling safe and being at ease, where defensive strategies can switch off, allowing the neural circuits that support rest and recuperation. If the physiology of the body is set to defend, the ability to relax, as well as the capacity for connection and expansive experience, is lost; the 'older' reptilian brain takes over to ensure survival, where behaviour reflects 'fight, flight or freeze'.

When Stephen Porges (2017) formulated the Polyvagal Theory to explain the neurobiology behind how 'our psychological, physical and behavioural responses are dependent on our physiological state' (p.47), he coined the term 'neuroception' (p.19), which refers to that part of the autonomic nervous system that is always online, evaluating risk to ensure survival.

Any perception of threat, however minute or unconscious, kicks off a physiological response where the capacity for relaxation, creativity and connection diminishes. Porges suggests through his theory that 'feeling safe is dependent on unique cues in the environment and in our relationships…that promote health and feelings of love and trust' (p.43). Many of the cues that reinforce feeling safe come from facial expression, tone of voice, gestures and posture – an evolution of the nervous system that enabled humans to turn off defensive mechanisms and live and work together in order to survive and flourish. A teacher's expression, vocal tone, movement and manner directly influence the ability to relax and experience the space as a safe haven.

Temperature also affects physiology – when the body is cold it tenses and shivers to produce heat, stimulating the nervous system through the production of adrenaline and other activating hormones. Ensure that there are plenty of blankets and that the temperature is comfortable when practising Restorative Yoga – not too hot or cold. Wear warm clothes that cover up the extremities when practising in order to be able to relax.

Bright lights and loud sounds are also highly stimulating. In the sanctuary of the space keep lights dim, but not too dark to navigate props. Avoid playing music in a Restorative class out of respect for the transforming power of stillness and space. If used at all, choose music that is spacious, austere and quieting.

In the end, quietude and space form the nurturing environment of a Restorative class or practice, where feeling safe and at ease supports neural pathways that reinforce relaxation and connection. (More on this in Chapter 15, The Art of Teaching Restorative Yoga.)

Be methodical and steady

Slow, methodical and steady movement within a class or practice reinforces feeling safe, as well as the quiet, introspective nature of the practice. Graceful and mindful movement when stretching or placing the props supports the nervous system and the experience of fullness of being.

A teacher's movement, stance and presence become part of the scaffolding of a Restorative class, which offers space for deep transformation. A teacher's presence eventually merges into the wholeness of the experience, adding to the wider tapestry of stillness and space where demonstration, timing of instruction and adjustments are part of the experience of deep relaxation.

Getting a prop, placing it and settling into a Restorative pose is part of a *process* that lends itself to relaxation. Unhurried, measured movement necessary during the transitions between poses expresses the choreography of an empowered movement towards the state of relaxation.

Pause and savour stillness

Understanding the rejuvenating power of a pause can free the psyche for the transformative power of Restorative practice, where stillness becomes a means to take in subtlety. Permission to become still brings into relief the natural exchange between inhale and exhale, where movement and stillness exist in equal measure. Restorative practice presents a powerful listening inwards that recognizes this exchange – where movement and stillness dance together in a delicate embrace.

Tasting stillness allows an appreciation for a dynamic wholeness that includes both activity and rest. Regularly practising Restorative Yoga redefines cultural misconceptions regarding work and rest and supports a wider shift in perception inclusive of practices that are deeply felt, and which encourage 'being' in balance with 'doing'.

Lie down and invert

A powerful cue to the nervous system, and one we use a lot in the Restorative practice, lying down begins a shift of the physiology towards relaxation. Lying down is restful for the heart as it no longer has to pump blood up to the head against the force of gravity. In addition, lying down or inverting (where the heart is higher than the head) stimulates the baroreflex, slowing the heart beat, lowering blood pressure and releasing muscular tension. When the baroreceptors register increased pressure in the neck from the shift in direction of blood flow towards the head, it initiates the relaxation response and quiets the brain.[3]

Lying prone on the front of the body can add to the relaxation response by enabling the power of a back body breath, which extends all the way down to the bottom tip of the lungs. When combined with the baroreflex, a soft and deep back body breath supports the physiology in the shift to 'rest and digest'. Note: lying on the side offers an option when unable to lie prone or supine.

---

3   Roger Cole Yoga (7 February, 2017) Restorative Yoga – How to use the baroreflex to relax more deeply: www.youtube.com/watch?v=NEpgS8utzu8&feature=emb_title. In this short YouTube clip, Roger very helpfully explains the science behind baroreceptors and why they do what they do.

Stay awhile

Longer holdings in the Restorative postures re-calibrate the nervous system, allowing time for a downshift into a slower, more nurturing mode. Depending on the posture, a pose can be held for anywhere between 5 and 30 minutes. In the arc of a practice, a long *śavāsana* (without instruction) at the end of the practice ensures this deep physiological shift.

If someone is chronically stressed it can take considerably longer to experience the shift of the nervous system. Put under stressful conditions for long enough, the nervous system will ramp itself up to operate at a faster pace and *stay there*. In order to remain in a mobilized state, energy may be redirected from other systems not central to survival such as digestion and reproduction, and this can lead to a health crisis and chronic illness. Longer holdings offer the time needed to shift gears, soften and rejuvenate.

Cultivate present moment awareness and the felt sense

Coming into present moment awareness offers an opening into 'the now' with all its subsequent sensations and layered experience; it serves as an anchor in time where past and future dissolve into the vibrancy of the present. The present state reveals what is happening and *felt* within the body's physiology, as well as in the psyche where thoughts, emotions, history and hope make up the emotional realm of self and identity.

Interoception refers to this ability to feel the inner sensations of the body, particularly with regard to what's happening in the autonomic nervous system (i.e. physiological state – fight, flight or rest). Stephen Porges (2017, p.15) defines it from the point of view of Polyvagal Theory as a 'process describing both conscious feelings and unconscious monitoring of bodily processes by the nervous system' as well as sensing changes in physiological state dependent on the two-way dialogue between body and brain. Bessel van der Kolk (2014, p.206) elaborates that it's possible to access and influence the reptilian brain (that oversees the survival response) through the medial pre-frontal cortex (that part of the brain that oversees self-awareness and the *felt sense*) and 'befriend' what is going inside.

In Restorative Yoga, time afforded in the postures allows space to inhabit the body and feel into what is present, noticing what is going on and taking steps to support this shift from sympathetic to parasympathetic mode. By paying attention to what is happening – an open listening that discerns state

– a conscious natural breath and softening can help move the body and mind towards homeostatic balance where relaxation or social engagement is possible.

In terms of practice, this means focusing on the felt sense of: the breath – its texture, flow, location and rhythm; the heart 'space' – its beat, rhythm, pace and emotional tone; the blood – its flow, circulation, warmth/coolness (of extremities) and its internal sound and sense; the muscles – their tonality, tension and patterns of holding and release; the digestion – literally and figuratively, its process of breaking down and taking in, felt both physically and emotionally; and the skin – its sensations of coolness and warmth, texture, moisture and sense of permeability. All these spaces and places embody physiological and symbolic aspects that regulate state.

By cultivating the ability to discern the different sensations within the body and being, the experiential sense of being alive – its wonder, depth and joy – can powerfully shift the nervous system towards balance. Relaxation arises from a deeply *felt* experience, acknowledged and processed.

PROPS – A DEFINING CHARACTERISTIC OF RESTORATIVE YOGA

Prop (noun) – something that props or sustains. *Prop* (verb) – to support by placing something under or against (Merriam-Webster online dictionary 2021).

Central to the practice, props offer support and comfort, encouraging the relaxation response. In addition, prop management and placement impact the flow and efficacy of a sequence, and can be approached with consideration and care to facilitate an inward experience.

Props adjust the body in different ways. A new bolster has a robustness that an old bolster lacks. Yet the older bolster offers softness and comfort like a well-worn pair of jeans. A buckwheat bolster moulds to the body, but sometimes can be too hard. But it can also serve as a grounding weight on top of the body. A prop can shift the whole dynamic and feel of a pose and influence the choices made when setting up a pose or crafting a sequence.

A student and friend of mine, who also teaches Restorative Yoga, once compared the aftermath of a practice to the state of disarray and dishevelment after a long-haul flight. I rather think she nailed it. Indeed, the prolific use of the props throughout the practice means the tidying up after the Restorative is in fact part of the process. To mindfully fold the blankets and place the bolsters and bricks back in their place reflects a settled and ordered mind. Taking care and moving slowly after the practice expresses the shift in physiological state.

Here's what's needed and why:

- *Bolsters* – cotton and/or buckwheat; a minimum of two per person. Bolsters provide the bulk of the prop foundation. One bolster goes a long way towards supporting the body in the way that is needed. It minimizes the number of props and the need to fold blankets. That said, a bolster can be seen as 'crude'. It doesn't allow for differences in bodies, and depending on its texture and composition – firm, soft, cotton or buckwheat – the nature of a bolster can deeply impact the body and nervous system. Generally speaking, a bolster should be firm but soft. It provides a stable structural support with a yielding tonality that allows for rest.

  I always get asked what kind of bolster is best for Restorative Yoga. It depends on what you are doing. Having a range of options is helpful. A rectangular cotton bolster is best for the spine; a round, full bolster works well for the back of the knees; a buckwheat bolster is great for snuggling up against the body or putting on top of the body as weight. The most practical bolsters have a handle on the top – this helps to pull the prop into the ideal placement. Finally, never throw away an old bolster. These are like gold when it comes to comfort and support. I've used the bolsters in my local class for 15 years and they've finally reached their perfect state. Just wash the covers!

- *Blankets* – both firm cotton and fleece; a minimum of two to four per person. Blankets can be folded in such a way as to fit into the body and can be seen as a more refined support than a bolster. That said, it requires presence of mind to fold the blanket in the right way and strategically place it where it needs to go. Usually, a firm cotton blanket works best for gross structural support, while the soft and warm fleece blankets work well for scrunching up and pressing into small places with curves, such as the head and neck, lumbar spine, flanks of the legs and edges of the feet.

  Sometimes, the soft and warm feel of the fleece blanket may be exactly what's needed to relax, while the strategically placed weight of a folded blanket offers comfort and grounding. Err on the side of more blankets in a practice. Their versatility and function are key in creating a nurturing, supportive and welcoming space.

- *Foam blocks* – flat and rectangular; a minimum of four per person. I sometimes think of the foam blocks as being like Lego – building blocks that when put together create a unique infrastructure of support. I particularly like 'angling' the foam blocks to meet the line of the legs such as in *supta baddha koṇāsana*, where holding the legs up allows the groins to soften down. There is a firmness to the block, and yet a softness that cradles. The wideness offers more support against the pull of gravity, and the composition of the foam blocks has a warmer tone, meeting the body with kindness. If foam blocks aren't available, the ever-resourceful blanket can be rolled, folded or scrunched to meet the need.

- *Cork brick* – one to two per person. I say cork and not wood, although if I had a wood brick I'd make use of it too. The cork is lighter and poses less risk of inadvertent and reverberating mishaps! There is nothing more disturbing during or after a Restorative practice than a wood brick clamouring down onto a hard floor – the expression 'jumping out of my skin' comes to mind – and then all that work to shift the physiology is lost in the 'fright' of the unexpected clap of sound.

  I particularly like rolling carefully across the edges of a brick to release patterns of holding in places like the rim of the skull or base of the pelvis. The firm and 'edgy' nature of this prop can release tension in the muscles and fascia that meet the brick's edges or faces. Bricks can also be used in different ways to support the limbs and in lieu of foam blocks.

- *Strap* – wide with square buckle; one per person (two is even better for certain stretches). (Don't bother with 'd-rings' or round-shaped buckles.) As strange as it may sound, the body is strapped in place in Restorative Yoga in order to lend support and allow release. Ease in getting into and out of the strap in the various postures becomes important for maintaining an even tone. The 'Pune' strap, as designed by Iyengar, allows for a pulling back which easily releases the buckle – a useful escape mechanism. In addition, the strap needs to be extra-long in order to perform certain stretches that require 'looping', and wide to offer more comfort against the skin.

  Finally, I always cover 'Strap 101' in my Restorative trainings. If the buckle is improperly secured, it will either break the buckle over time or simply won't catch, an undesirable and often agitating outcome. This means learning how the strap works and taking the time in practice or class to discover and master the magnificence of its simplicity.

- *Sticky mat* – one per person. Picking a mat is a personal thing. The only thing to consider here would be the cushioning factor. When lying on the floor for longer holdings, the firmness of the floor can make itself known. Double-up sticky mats so there is more cushion and/or add a folded blanket on top for further cushioning and warmth. Always come back to what makes the practice space cosy and inviting.

- *Sandbags* – rectangular with handles; two per person. Sandbags offer a way to strategically weight the body and ground it. Putting the weight on limbs, belly or even forehead initiates a type of release both physically and mentally in a way that dramatically shifts the physiology. While it's called a 'sand' bag, often rice or gravel is used. The ideal weight of a sandbag is anywhere from 5 to 10 lb.[4]

  Positioning a sandbag constitutes an art. For the hips, angle the sand bag inwardly to soften the groin, placing it just below the hip joint. Sometimes a sandbag may be too heavy – you will know because it will either feel uncomfortable, or a limb will feel as if it's starting to fall asleep. In this case, use a lighter sandbag, or a bolster or a folded blanket.

- *Eye pillows* – two per person. Weight on the forehead helps to shift the thinking mind to a state of rest. When placed on the eyes, it settles eye movement associated with an outward focus. Sometimes, when we are afraid, the eyes stay wide open, indicating that the physiology is geared towards fight or flight. A simple eye pillow strategically placed can break this pattern of response and shift the state towards relaxation.

  I prefer a double eye pillow approach – one placed across the brow, and the other tipped off its lower edge and onto the bridge of the nose. This arrangement blocks light and adds the necessary weight without placing it on the eyeball itself, which for some can be uncomfortable. It is always best to check in with people *before* placing the eye pillow – for some, closing the eyes can make them feel unsafe. It's fine to allow students the choice to keep the eyes softly open if this is more comfortable. A shawl draped across the eyes is also an option.

- *Chair* – metal with no back or a bar on the front legs; one per person (two works best for tall folks). While any chair can be made to work, the

---

4   Recommended by Richard Rosen. He's partial to a 5 lb weight on the belly.

metal ones adapted for yoga work best. There are ones designed for taller people too. That said, if you are smaller, in some cases it's best to build a 'bolster chair' to the height that suits.

A final note about props…clean them regularly! There is nothing more off-putting than coming to a class or practice and discovering an unpleasant smell emanating from your bolster or blanket. Whether it's your own or you're a teacher at a studio that provides the props, put in place a washing regime that refreshes and reassures. In this case, cleanliness is definitely next to godliness!

PROP 'LIGHT' PRACTICE AND IMPROVISING AT HOME

As stated above, props are a defining characteristic of Restorative practice. Without them, it's simply not a Restorative class; rather a relaxation or gentle yoga class. That said, there are certain postures that can be adapted to what I call 'prop light', such as: accordion folding a blanket and placing it underneath the spine; raising the pelvis up on a foam block or blanket with a strap around the thighs; or placing a brick as weight on the solar plexus. If I find myself at a studio that has only a few props, I work out what I can do, sacrificing the extra frills that make the practice especially Restorative. What's the minimum? Probably a couple of blankets, a foam block or brick and a belt.

Teaching Restorative classes online also requires improvisation with regard to props. Students may not have two bolsters, four foams, two bricks, four blankets, a belt and an eye pillow just lying around their house… In which case, there are a number of ways to use everyday household items as props. For example, books can serve as blocks. You can accordion fold blankets into the height of a bolster or fold a pillow length-ways and wrap it in a blanket to hold it together, tying it with belts. Pillows from couches are excellent underneath knees and the head to lend support. The belt off a dressing gown or house coat makes for a great substitute belt as it is long. Cushions from the couch often work well as a uniquely shaped bolster or even a padded weight on the front of the body.

In the end, the practice can be adjusted to meet the need. Rule of thumb… don't allow any major joints to hang against gravity for too long. Find something suitable that offers a sense of support. Otherwise the body will brace to hold itself against the force of gravity, which stimulates the nervous system, defeating the goal of the practice.

Chapter 5

Community and Connection

If I said that my love for you was
like the spaces between the notes of a wren's song,
would you understand?

The Unwinding by Jackie Morris (2020)

A good friend of mind once described her experience of a Restorative Yoga class as oddly comforting. The experience of resting on the floor in semi-darkness, side by side with complete strangers, made her feel part of a something remarkable – what emerged for her was a profound sense of belonging.

Tyler VanderWeele (2020), Director of the Human Flourishing Program at Harvard University, presents research that shows coming together with others in shared purpose expresses an important aspect of human beings flourishing. At the end of a Restorative class, an undeniable softness of facial expression reveals delicate strands of interrelationship strengthened through a process of space, release and renewal. A fine tapestry of connection, compelling in its vividness and colour, opens the heart, giving rise to a collective joy.

While people come to a Restorative class for different reasons, there exists a powerful alchemy in community that comforts and heals. Simply put, coming together in unified purpose magnifies the end result. A quiet presence of distilled joy reflected in slow movement and body language speaks of trust and the transforming power of human connection.

In a world that at times can seem fractious and disjointed, a Restorative class offers an oasis of calm and protection, where people can come together and experience the beauty of stillness and space. A balm to a frazzled nervous system, a class reaffirms the truth of how physiology impacts the ability to meaningfully connect, as well as the interwoven nature of community, presence and joy.

Sometimes, Restorative practice can reveal underlying agitation or irritability. The power of stillness becomes like a mirror that reflects back the fractures of self normally hidden underneath movement and activity. It is at these times when the embrace of community supports healing. While the practice unfolds through individual enquiry, the community offers a collective sanctuary where inner challenges can be met and overcome in silent solidarity.

Practices that ask us to slow down, become still and feel without reacting are described as 'revolutionary' by inspired thinker and leader Margaret Wheatley in her seminal book *Who Do We Choose to Be? Facing Reality, Claiming Leadership and Restoring Sanity* (2017). She describes these types of practices as 'restorative'. While she isn't specifically referring to Restorative Yoga, her insight is helpful in understanding the power of the Restorative work: 'They [practices that require becoming still and listening] are processes that reawaken our powers of cognition, reinstitute thinking, and redirect our attention to one another.' She goes further to say that as a 'collective of minds, we see more clearly' (p.198).

She poses an important question, 'How do we create islands of sanity that sustain our best human qualities?' (p.18). When I first heard this expression, 'islands of sanity', I immediately thought about the nurturing environment of a Restorative class, where practices that settle and nurture reveal the best part of human 'being'.

When I reflect back on my own experience of yoga, and the extraordinary teachers who have enlivened my understanding, there is one teaching that stands out. It has to do with taking responsibility, and what this means: taking responsibility for my state; making the effort to reflect and consider how my actions may impact others; and a conscious recognition of the interconnected fabric of being where a kind word and smile can lighten someone's load and summon joy. It's worth noting how the word responsibility can be seen as response-ability – the ability to respond – which only transpires when physiological state allows. Restorative practice helps cultivate a state of being where 'responding' is actually possible.

The culture in a Restorative class exudes a warm and steadfast welcome – a safe haven for coming together and connecting without fear – where distinctions of class, race, gender or sexual preference disappear amid a common need to relax and feel connection. While practice is quiet and individual, it is also communal, and that is part of its power. Practice teaches a new definition of responsibility that engenders nourishment, protection and healing in community; where the impulse to uplift arises from the experience of connection and commonality.

Again, inspired by Wheatley (2017), a Restorative class becomes a radical act of 'transcendence' especially in fragmented and fragile times. It affirms equilibrium and amplifies the energy of connection where resting back (literally) transforms the finitude of a moment into an experience of the infinite – love speaks in the quiet space of the heart's connection. There is space to experience, feel and embrace human 'being' in all its inter-connective depth. To come together in community and…rest. Restorative Yoga cultivates a stable mindset that allows the *choice* of connection and, ultimately, wellbeing – which speaks to our long history in yoga that seeks first to unify inwardly, then outwardly.

To practise Restorative Yoga inspires the question: What is truly important? Self or Other? Or both as two sides of the same coin?

Chapter 6

Ātmavicāra

SELF-ENQUIRY

There is a long history of self-enquiry as a practice in yoga. It says in the *Aparokṣānabhūti*, an 8th–9th-century text attributed to *Adi Śaṅkarācārya* and translated by Swami Vimuktananda, 'Knowledge is not brought about by any other means than self-enquiry, just as an object is nowhere perceived without the help of light.' An indispensable practice of discernment, *ātmavicāra* or self-enquiry serves as a *process* of questioning and illumination; it embraces deep contemplation of the self (what I describe as 'fullness of being') as a means to invoke its experience. John Grimes (1996, p.69) translates *ātmavicāra* as literally, 'enquiry into the nature of the Self'.

The process of self-enquiry necessarily involves identifying ways of thinking or viewing that serve as obstacles on a path dedicated to liberation. This usually begins with a quintessential question, such as, 'Who am I?' It continues by asking questions that tap into inner wisdom and penetrate through the layers of unconscious delusions and projections regarding self and others. The process of questioning uncovers the true nature of reality beyond the thinking mind with its many judgements and opinions. This contemplative self-examination reveals habitual patterns and tendencies that block the experience of fullness of being. Referred to in yoga as *saṁskāras*, these separating tendencies operate as binding subterranean scripts that influence perception, behaviour and state, and ultimately the experience of deep connection.

Shining the light of awareness through a process of questioning can elicit an experiential epiphany, an 'aha' moment of recognition and release. Just as light disperses shadow, self-enquiry and awareness can illumine and attenuate self-limiting narratives and behaviours. Once a *saṁskāra* is seen and known, it loses its grip – there is space to choose a different response and move towards the experience of wholeness, or liberation.

In *Roots of Yoga*, Mallinson and Singleton (2017) point out that the original renunciant ascetics, progenitors of modern yoga, held ideas of liberation that involved ending the cycle of rebirth (*saṃsāra*) and karma-driven suffering. But what does liberation actually mean from the seat of a 21st-century yogi? I can't really comment about rebirth, and there's a complexity to the notion of karma that can be highly misunderstood. What I do know is that I can change the frame of perception by regularly asking questions which challenge assumptions and beliefs. I can engage in an intentional process of questioning that results in being freed from a pattern of behaviour or thought that results in suffering. In this way, liberation comes through small unexpected moments of revelation: how I am responsible for my suffering through what I am thinking; how awareness enables choice; and how the *experience* of a moment can offer depth, joy and meaning. That, to me, is liberation or freedom.

Restorative Yoga offers a useful means for engaging in contemplative practice in the spirit of *ātmavicāra*. Its slow and felt nature allows time and space for enquiry. In his book *Exquisite Love*, Bill Mahony (2014, p.158) translates *ātmavicāra* literally as a 'movement into the Self'. The Restorative poses afford time for a conscious movement towards self, a state of integration, that is *felt* through relaxation. I call this type of enquiry embodied presence – sensing inwards, feeling and experiencing the rejuvenating fullness of one's own being, which 'embodies' a wider intent to know the nature of self and being. (More on this in Chapter 7, Embodied Presence.)

Asking specific questions through writing a journal and contemplation presents another way to practise self-enquiry, smoothing the way for the depth of Restorative practice. It helps to reveal and penetrate through habitual impressions or *saṃskāras* in order to experience one's essential nature. Practising this method of enquiry directly investigates patterns of thinking, concepts and cultural imprints that may interfere with the ability to relax and dive deep. It cultivates the stability of mind and presence necessary to source inner wisdom, and serves as a powerful way to navigate the discomfort that can arise when becoming still and seeking rest. Perceptions of lack or disempowering self-beliefs are rooted out, and self-knowledge is applied in a practical way for the sake of lived experience and lasting joy. This can't happen while there are unconscious embedded narratives toxic to the state of happiness.

THE PROCESS OF CONTEMPLATION

Listed below are a series of questions designed to provoke thought and enquire into beliefs and assumptions with regard to relaxation and rest; they provide a means to access inner wisdom. It involves a two-part process of enquiry and contemplation. For this practice, you will need a quiet space, a journal, pen and some uninterrupted time. The questions intentionally overlap in order to elicit and highlight insight. Pick one group and work with it for a few days. Don't rush. Rather, explore your thoughts on the matter and notice the physical response of your body, as well as the emotional response of your mind.

I take inspiration from Julia Cameron's, *The Artist's Way* (1992).[1] In this seminal book on spirituality through the practice of creativity, she shares a method of writing whatever comes to mind as a basic tool to access creative power – what she calls 'morning pages'. It encourages handwriting your thoughts without censor. The process described here is somewhat similar and also inspired from my experience of study and contemplation at the ashram. First, it involves answering a series of questions that engage the mind in self-reflection. Second, it involves asking a quintessential question in order to access the deeper wellspring of wisdom within, and seeing what arises.

To begin, select the body of questions you'd like to engage with, and write them down in your journal. Then, spend time unabashedly answering the questions, writing whatever comes up in your mind. Don't censor. No one else will read this. Get all the thoughts out of your mind and down on the paper. When you've 'downloaded' all your thoughts, then and only then, put down your pen and set the journal aside.

Next, consider the quintessential question. Close your eyes and…breathe. Wait. In stillness. Sense the heart area or the feel of the breath's ebb and flow. Empty the mind of its thoughts and listen inwards to your being. Pose the quintessential question to the wellspring of wisdom within and see what inspiration arises. After sitting in stillness with the question for a while, write down any wisdom that may bubble up to the surface of awareness. Recognize and trust that

---

1   Julia Cameron's book, *The Artist's Way: A Spiritual Path to Higher Creativity*, was a lifeline during my twenties; it profoundly shifted my views regarding creativity, strength and how to access inner wisdom. I found myself challenging fear at all levels. Combined with the intensive practices and learning of yoga at the ashram, it was a truly transformative time. The morning pages were instrumental in embedding self-enquiry as a means to uncover and see things as they are. Julia explains her process of morning pages more in depth in her book from pages 9 to 18.

there is inner knowledge and insight waiting to be sourced. If nothing arises, continue to work with the question(s) over a longer period of time.

This type of self-enquiry encompasses a lifetime process of questioning that investigates limiting narratives/behaviours that interfere with the state of connection. The process of questioning and presence initiates revelation that arises from an *inner* wellspring. Consistent practice of self-enquiry invites ongoing insight and understanding. Revisiting the same questions can be interesting. Insight sparkles like a multi-faceted diamond; light and position can change the angle of perception bringing forth new knowledge and wisdom.

QUESTIONS

Answer the 'journaling questions' first engaging with your mind; then put your pen down, become still and contemplate the 'quintessential question' with your being…

————

Journaling questions: Do you find it hard to pause, settle and turn inwards? Why? Describe what happens. How/where do you it feel in the body? What thoughts arise? What repetitive statements occur? What happens at the soul level?

————

- *Quintessential question:* Why do I find it so hard to stop and pause?

————

Journaling questions: What comes up when you consider rest and relaxation as a part of your life? Write down your initial thoughts. Write down any judgements that may arise. Reflect on your history of rest and relaxation. What is a defining characteristic?

- *Quintessential question:* What comes up from deep inside, when I try to rest and relax?

————

Journaling questions: Do you feel that you do enough? Do you hold guilt around the notion of 'not doing enough'? Explore the concept of 'what is enough?' in your journal, and consider your relationship to it.

————

- *Quintessential question:* What will allow me to feel I am enough, just as I am?

———————

Journaling questions: What is your pattern with regard to work and rest? Is it balanced? If you could change your pattern, what would it look like?

- *Quintessential question:* Why do I find it so hard to experience balance?

———————

Journaling questions: When can you first remember having the thought that it was lazy to not do anything? Where do you think this notion came from? How has this impacted your life?

- *Quintessential question:* Who am I, if I'm not busy doing something?

———————

Journaling questions: Have you ever had the thought that Restorative Yoga isn't 'real' yoga? What is 'real' yoga? How has this belief about this style of practising affected your experience of yoga? Of living?

- *Quintessential question:* What is the real value of yoga for me?

———————

Journaling questions: Describe the way you respond to stress – the pattern in the body, within the mind. Look more closely at your pattern of response in stressful situations – the repetitive thoughts involved with the pattern. Is there a common theme?

- *Quintessential question:* How can I let go of my stressful reactions?

———————

Journaling questions: How do you see yourself in relationship with the world? Describe the way you interact and feel with regard to life and living. Is there a dominant tone? Is there anything that holds you back from living fully? What's truly important to you?

- *Quintessential question:* What is the true purpose of my life?

———————

Journaling questions: 'What is the pattern that connects?' Describe your feeling,

———————

experience and understanding of this statement by Gregory Bateson (1979, p.8). What is your experience of the state of interconnection?

- *Quintessential question:* What is my essential nature, beyond what I think, do or feel?

SUMMARY OF PART I

Restorative Yoga has evolved from the long and rich history of the yoga tradition, finding its modern form through the assiduous efforts of B.K.S. Iyengar. Within an environment of calm, quiet and simplicity, this style of yoga enables a downshift of the nervous system into deep relaxation, which removes fatigue and rejuvenates. By consciously slowing down, grounding and taking the support of the breath, Restorative Yoga promotes stability of mind and a sense of wellbeing. A refreshed perception amplifies the ability to connect. Nervous system health, propping the body and stillness distinguish it from other introspective styles. The power of community and self-enquiry further deepen the transformational power of Restorative Yoga.

Part II

PRESENCE

To settle into the texture of a moment opens the door into the space of infinite being revealing an inner landscape the essence of which is joyful.

Chapter 7

———

Embodied Presence

In the beginning was non-existence.
From this, truly, existence emerged.
By itself, it made a body for itself.
Therefore, it is called 'the well-made'.
That is the essence of existence.
Tasting that essence, one becomes joyful.
Who could live, who could breathe,
if that essence did not exist as joy?
For it is that essence that causes joy.

Taittirīya Upaniṣad 2.7.1[1]

WHAT DOES EMBODIED PRESENCE MEAN?

Presence is an interesting word. As a noun, the Merriam-Webster online dictionary (2021) refers to it as 'the fact or condition of being present'. More and more, I've heard it being used as a verb to describe the action of resting back into the fullness of a moment…to enter into the experience of fullness of being.

This is my experience of Restorative Yoga. It serves as a means to dive deep inside and feel into the very fabric of body, psyche and being – to attend to

———

1   Translation by Bill Mahony. Bill has an inspired touch when translating from Sanskrit to English, and he shares the meaning and subtlety of this verse with such *joy*. His careful choice of words enlivened by his dedicated study and direct experience conveys the yoga tradition's teachings with depth and beauty. I am grateful to know him these past 20 years and thank him for sharing his knowledge and insight so clearly and freely.

———

bodily sensations and feelings as a way to connect to the profound aliveness within a moment, extracting its fullness and sourcing the underlying joy of being. As a yogi, I view this process as one of seeking to know the very nature of who and what I am in a way that is felt and transmitted through experience, rather than through words or ideas.

As a present moment endeavour, the practice of embodied presence serves as a means to dip into the experience of what is *already happening*. Not in the past, or in the future, but right now in this body – through this form – the end result being transcendent and ecstatic. This is essentially a Tantric concept. In the words of Georg Feuerstein (1998, p.60), 'The Tantric approach is to see all life experiences as the play of the same One.' He also elaborates on Tantra's goal as being similar to all Indic liberation teachings: '…to move beyond all suffering and discover the indescribable bliss of Being' (p.59).

I'd like to highlight a concept advanced in Tantra that enlivens Restorative practice and further elucidates the feel of embodied presence – that the body itself is divine. Tantra diverged from the earlier ascetic traditions which viewed the body as something to be renounced. Rather, the body became the means to experience the cosmos itself in all its glory (Mallinson and Singleton 2017).

Along with this Tantric way of viewing reality and practising yoga, one of my favourite verses that describes this notion of microcosm/macrocosm comes from an earlier text, the *Chāndogya Upaniṣad* (8.1.2) translated by Olivelle (2008, p.167): 'As vast as the space here around us is this space within the heart, and within it are contained both the earth and the sky, both fire and wind, both the sun and the moon, both lightning and stars.'

What is this 'space within the heart'? To enquire into subjective experience through the layers of embodiment sourcing 'the body as divine' points to a radical shift of perception: from the stance of 'separate from' to 'intrinsically part of' the universe. To seek and know this ineffable essence at the heart of human 'being' has been the focus of yogic practices described through various ontologies (models of existence) over the millennia.

Restorative Yoga embodies this type of enquiry, affirming its place in the evolution of the yoga tradition. The introspective work demands interest in the inner experience, as well as the nature of consciousness itself: to 'presence' fullness of being hidden in the centre of self and soul.

Embodied presence refers then to a profound enquiry into the sensory nature of 'being' fully felt and savoured. It reveals the 'completeness' of an unfolding moment as *experienced* through the senses. It is a conscious movement towards one's essence beyond individual notions – a hearkening to the universal. We can engage in this type of enquiry as a means to tap the wisdom latent in every cell of the body, and access an underlying state of abiding joy, the goal of practice.

A ROADMAP INWARDS

It's helpful to have a road map for this movement towards essence. Yoga offers a few. I often work with one from nondual Śaiva Tantra as described by Hareesh Wallis (2013) in his book, *Tantra Illuminated*; he calls this map the Tantrik Five-Layered Self.[2] Combined with a physical practice, it can help navigate the complexity of human 'being' by providing a progressive structure for enquiry and understanding.

The layers of being move from coarse to subtle, the first layer being the physical body itself called *deha*.[3] Exploring the felt sense of the body through skin, blood, muscles, sinew, fascia, bones and so on offers a tangible way to know and sense the body itself – to feel into the form as a first step on the inward journey.

The second layer, considered the 'thickest' layer of being, can be thought of as the psyche – the mind/emotion layer known as *citta*. It includes the mind's movement through thoughts and emotions; the sense of individual identity and notions of ownership. *Citta* also includes the intellect – the ability to discern and choose. It's also here that the structure of the yogic or subtle body resides (i.e. *cakras* and *nāḍis*).[4]

The third layer known as *prāṇa* – the vital energy layer intimately connected with the breath – enlivens the body–mind layers. More subtle in form than mind, emotions and intellect, the vital energy of *prāṇa* flows through the subtle structures of the second layer like electricity flows through circuits. *Prāṇa* serves as the dynamic energy which connects the body and mind, enabling its function. All of nature resonates with this vital energy; it goes beyond the sense of the individual, which is why it's considered more subtle.

Beyond *prāṇa*, the fourth layer, *śūnya* or void, expresses as transcendent stillness, space and silence. I feel this layer becomes prominent within Restorative practice. It's a settling inwards into the feel of spacious being where the

2 Wallis chooses to spell Tantrik with a 'k'. He speaks more on his reasons for this in *Tantra Illuminated*.

3 Wallis mentions that some sources add a peripheral layer of 'stuff' or the material things that surround us – I chuckle at this. In Restorative Yoga, it's the immense pile of props!

4 The subtle body came into its full expression within Tantra.

mind becomes still and there is deep rest. This layer can be experienced as a type of 'deep sleep'. When I fall into this state, I come out surprised – where have I been?! I know I haven't actually fallen asleep, I've just simply disappeared and there is no sense of time passing. I come back feeling refreshed.

But this isn't the final destination. We eventually enter a realm that is not really a layer at all. It exists beyond all layers and simultaneously pervades through them as them: we arrive at the centre of being known as *cit* or *saṃvit* – a state of absolute consciousness or awareness,[5] a timeless state of pure being ever unfolding, supremely blissful and undivided. This is the beauty of Tantra as a philosophy and why I gravitate towards this model – it emphasizes joy as essence.

This particular roadmap offers an artful and accessible way to tap into and sense the different layers of being when turning inwards, whether during *śavāsana*, a sequence of Restorative poses or for meditation. It offers a conceptualization for conscious embodiment and explores the premise that we are more than just the body or thoughts and feelings – where joy or bliss exists *as* the core of being, suffusing and pervading all layers.

The vast and varied inner landscape of conscious human embodiment contains colour, contrast and tremendous beauty, just like that of the outer landscape. Restorative Yoga gives time and space for the exploration of this rich inner world, starting with that which is most tangible…the physical body, and from there moving *inwards*.

Embodied presence engenders a movement towards wholeness and establishes interrelationship as a principle of existence. This movement inwards, sensing and feeling, cultivates the focus and subtlety of perception needed to discern and experience essence. For me, this is the reason I practise yoga: to bring about a subtle shift that allows an experience of fullness arising from within, where a sense of wellbeing resonates as the state of connection.

Nora Bateson (2016, p.17), in her book *Small Arcs of Larger Circles,* shares passionately, '…there is something holding all of this together, all of us together. There is an alive order that we are within that is within us.' Restorative Yoga offers a means to realize this extraordinary and simple truth.

---

5   This blog by Wallis is helpful in explaining more fully the Five-Layered Self in relationship to the koshas. https://hareesh.org/blog/2015/12/16/the-five-koshas-and-the-five-layered-self-a-comparison.

MORE ON THE JOY OF BEING AND RESTORATIVE YOGA

The enquiry-based nature of Restorative practice points people back to their own *felt* experience and removes the worry of being right or wrong or having a 'perfect' pose. There is permission to feel into all aspects of embodiment and essence without censure, where curiosity inspires investigation. Curiosity and the state of balance go hand-in-hand, creating a foundation for the experience of joy.

Coming from the Latin root *cūra*, which means 'care' in the sense of taking pains (Barnhart 1988, p.243), Restorative Yoga offers an empowered space for taking time to be curious and listen inwards. This process of self-discovery through embodied presence allows meaning-making free from outer influences and lends itself to an unfolding sense of purpose in relation to the whole. Sociologist Aaron Antonovsky (1987) refers to this as the sense of coherence – feeling part of a wider structure of meaning which is necessary for wellbeing and worth cultivating.

Embodied presence helps to establish these inner pathways of connection. Turning inwards becomes a navigating force for tapping into essence, or fullness of being. Postures offer a means for discovering and knowing at a cellular level what Gregory Bateson (1979, p.8) described as 'the pattern that connects'. This can only happen when there is time and the physiological state to lean into the nature of self and being. Posing a broad question at the beginning of practice, such as 'Who am I?' or 'What is my essential nature?' and letting the question sit in the unfolding space of embodied presence over the course of a practice can initiate a *felt* truth that transforms perception, enabling the ability to feel the state of interconnection.

A verse from the *Taittirīya Upaniṣad* (2.7.1) shared at the beginning of this chapter (and translated so beautifully by Bill Mahony) establishes a clear relationship between essence and joy. Non-existence suggests a state of pure being or essence prior to manifestation that resonates as joy. Existence refers to the body and manifest world as made up of that essence. One *sources* the other.

A Restorative practice allows time to explore this teaching by turning inwards through the layers of being and tasting essence, the nature of which is joy-*full*. The verse suggests that each human being embodies this essence and is, therefore, well made. To practise Restorative Yoga becomes a conscious dipping into the sense of self as whole and well-made. What a radical act! To renounce ways of thinking that self-limit and criticize; to reaffirm ones that honour and recognize the perfection that we already are.

Through this style of practice, stillness and space become associated with joy. Learning to savour a sense of spaciousness reclaims energy that has been caught in the form of self-limiting narratives, written in patterns of holding in the body. Root fears and tendencies can be safely released from their restrictive form back into essence – a merging that results in a state of deep connection. This merging can be experienced as a profound joy – an integration at the deepest layer of our being.

Time also seems to stop in Restorative Yoga as the preoccupation with outer matters recedes to an inner experience of peacefulness – where individual identity temporarily dissolves into the vibrancy and presence of a singular and infinite moment. Rejuvenation occurs by shifting the limited perception of form to the limitless aspect of 'being', nestled in the very heart of body and soul.

Restorative practice unfolds a powerful state of subjective experience, rejuvenating in its affirmation of wholeness and the joy of being. By tapping into this inner wellspring – niṣprapañca, 'never not there' – the body, mind and soul come together fulfilling yet another nuance in the meaning of yūj, or yoke, the root syllable in the translation of yoga, which embodies the state of connection.

RESTORATIVE OR MEDITATION: ARE THEY DIFFERENT?

I often get this question regarding the difference between Restorative Yoga and meditation. While the two practices are distinctly different in form, they overlap in common purpose – investigating the nature of self and being. Restorative Yoga can be helpful in preparing for meditation practice, facilitating the downshift of the nervous system so necessary for turning inwards.

Restorative Yoga emphasizes nervous system health and deep relaxation; meditation emphasizes an inner alertness that navigates the vicissitudes of the mind. In the end, both styles of yoga practice lead to the same destination – a deep absorption in essence and the joy of being.

FINAL WORDS

Much of the practice of embodied presence happens through the sensitivity and expression of the breath. Within the inner landscape, breath serves as a means to deeply feel and move towards the centre. It profoundly influences state and serves as a means to tap into a resonant sense of aliveness both energizing and transcendent.

Chapter 8

─────

The Breath as Teacher and Friend

The answers live in the lands of dreamers, between a breath and a breath, in open hearts and open hands.

The Unwinding by Jackie Morris (2020)

FIRST, MIDDLE AND LAST TEACHER

Breath flows in…the first act entering into the world – a powerful 'I am here!' of form and substance. Continuing in a tireless manner over the course of a lifetime, the breath's movement sustains, nourishes and comforts like a good friend. Breath flows out…the last act exiting this world – a powerful surrender into the great mystery beyond.

Breath – the first, middle and last teacher – can serve as a wise guide through every stage of life. Playing a central role in Restorative practices, it powerfully adjusts physiological state and provides a unique metronome for present moment awareness. Most of the time this ever-present rhythm sourcing all movement and activity isn't noticed, but it bears scrutiny. A 'defining practice' in pre-modern India, breath control was regarded by medieval yogis as a means of attaining the highest states of being (Mallinson and Singleton 2017, p.127). And yet, is 'control' really the right word? Or is it more like surfing a magnificent wave – a delicate balancing act of following and flowing with the power of nature expressed through the simple form of inhale, pause, exhale, pause?

─────

When the breath is made conscious – drawn out (*dīrgha*) and subtle (*sūkṣma*) as translated in Bryant's *Yoga Sūtras of Patañjali* (2009, p.290, II.50) – something extraordinary happens. The present moment expands into relief and vibrates with power. Breath becomes a potent teacher mapping the contours of the body, disclosing unnecessary tension, downshifting the nervous system and revealing the joy of being through its flow…and ebb. Breath symbolizes the power of life – its movement and stillness – from beginning, to middle, to end.

According to the yoga tradition, the very essence of life is contained within the breath, an enlivening force described as *prāṇa*, life-breath or the primary breath. It is responsible for the vital functions of the body and it pervades every particle of the universe, bestowing the gift of an animate world. Composed of two root words in Sanskrit, '*pra*' to bring forth and '*an*' to breathe, *prāṇa* expresses the creative power of life ever unfolding. Sometimes it's translated as energy, vitality or power (Rosen 2002).

In medieval yoga practice, *prāṇāyāma* refers to the control of the breath. In some texts the translation of '*āyāma*' means to extend. It was mostly considered a means to purify and prepare for the upward rise of this vital energy, result-ing in final liberation (Mallinson and Singleton 2017). Both the translation of *prāṇa* and the words breath 'control' imply an expansion to be approached with awareness, care and caution.

There is a parable from the *Chāndogya Upaniṣad* (5.1.6–15) translated by Olivelle (2018, p.137) which conveys the power of *prāṇa*. In this story, the 'vital functions' of speech, sight, hearing, mind and breath compete to see who is the greatest. They go to their father Prajāpati for clarity and he says, 'The one, after whose departure the body appears to be in the worst shape, is the greatest among you.' One at a time they leave the body and come back. When it's time for breath to leave, the other vital functions realize their folly and beg breath to stay… Breath alone sustains life.

While formal *prāṇāyāma* practices have their place and purpose, I feel breath awareness offers a gentler approach that better supports the intent of Restorative practices. Looking back at the history of yoga, *prāṇāyāma* has been criticized for its difficulty (Mallinson and Singleton 2017), from the Buddha to Abhinavagupta, the brilliant 10th–11th-century Śaiva scholar and polymath. From my own personal experience, I have sometimes found the complexity and forcefulness of the different *prāṇāyāma* techniques to cause stress and anxiety; the simplicity of breath awareness can be equally effective in expanding a sense of vitality, resulting in renewal and awakening.

Breath awareness in this sense refers to consciously experiencing the breath's expression as a way to stay anchored in the present and release unnecessary tension – to encourage a free and easeful breath that is rejuvenating and healing. (More on this in Chapter 10, A Free and Easeful Breath.)

Through utilizing a conscious breath that is felt and followed, breath awareness serves as a process for feeling into self and being; it lends support to the natural expression of the breath without trying to manipulate it. Always moving and changing to meet the circumstances of the moment, a conscious breath offers a tangible way to feel into the body's shape, texture and response, helping to adjust state and release tension. Tuning in to the feel of the breath as it moves initiates a process which makes known that which is unconscious and releases that which is held. Like a good friend, the breath gently whispers to us what we need to hear.

During the quiet introspection of a Restorative pose, listening through the felt-sense of the breath reaffirms the innate connection of the body and mind. In Blandine Calais-Germain's book, *Anatomy of Breathing* (2006, p.13), she artfully describes the breath: 'It influences our actions and our emotions and at the same time is influenced by them. On the other hand it is an action that one can influence in a conscious, voluntary manner...' Highlighting this notion that the breath and mind are 'inextricably linked', Mallinson and Singleton (2017, p.132) identify several texts across the yoga tradition where steadiness of mind leads to the liberated state. When the breath flows freely in a balanced manner, it draws forth an evenness that soothes; a softness and sensitivity needed to dive deep into a sense of wholeness.

Moving with the power of a natural breath becomes a teacher of enormous value. Through the breath's measured grace, the ability to ascertain what is happening internally cultivates subtlety of perception. The body softens within the embrace of a Restorative posture; moving with the breath's rhythm, the mind finds succour. The inhale expands the form in exhilaration like a bird taking flight, the exhale provides a powerful release that enables a deep shift into abiding peacefulness.

Not only does the breath adjust the physiology towards balance, it also reveals what is present and provides the felt understanding of a unified experience. An ever-present resource, breath amplifies connection while simultaneously rejuvenating and nourishing. There is much to gain from exploring its depth, expression and splendour. It could be argued the breath is the only teacher, pulsing with the beauty of life captured in form.

BREATH AS A PATHWAY INWARDS

The practice of embodied presence utilizes the breath as a means to explore the landscape of being. It offers a navigating force for enquiring into the inner realms of conscious embodiment. By sensing the layers of being through the steady companionship of the breath, listening and feeling through its pulsation, thought diminishes, giving rise to the simple joy of being.

Breath also provides an anchor to a vibrant unfolding moment where the activity of doing evaporates into the resonant space of pure being. An anchor in a tumultuous sea of thoughts and emotions, breath provides a safe harbour within which to reclaim energy caught in stories. Dispelling toxic narratives that drain and diminish, it exists as the power of present moment awareness, pulsing with a tangible feeling of presence and fullness.

The breath's expression provides an interesting way to turn inwards and learn about the nature of conscious embodiment. There are four expressions of the breath which can serve as a helpful guide on the roadmap towards essence: inhale (*pūraka*), the pause at the depth of the inhale (*antara-kumbhaka*), exhale (*recaka*), and the pause at the end of the exhale (*bāhya-kumbhaka*). Each movement of the breath sourced in stillness offers a taste of the power of pure being which can be accessed through simple breath awareness.

Furthermore, when combined with the power of imagination, the breath can be visualized as currents of vital energy flowing through the body in ways that can rejuvenate, awaken and heal. In a restful Restorative posture, a combination of intent and imagery can help unlock the enlivening power of *prāṇa* contained within the breath's flow, sourcing the tradition's 'yogic' or subtle body as an integral part of the roadmap towards essence or centre.[1]

The totality of the breath's expression epitomizes the paradox at the heart of existence captured so beautifully in 'Burnt Norton' by T.S. Eliot (1944, p.5) as 'the still point of the turning world'. The inexorable flow of inhale and exhale arises from and returns to an ever-present stillness. As such, the breath provides a compelling focus for diving deep into embodiment as a means to investigate essence. A main focus in Restorative practice, the breath emanates fullness

---

1   Both Tantra and later *haṭhayoga* schools practised visualizing subtle pathways through the body in order to adjust the flow of *prāṇa*. They were particularly intent on raising *kuṇḍalinī*, the spiritual power coiled at the base of the spine, through the primary central channel called *suṣumnā nāḍi* in order to attain the highest reality (Mallinson and Singleton 2017, p.178).

of being where physiology and spirituality combine to heighten vitality and connection. Freeing the breath and attention are key.[2]

THE SPACE IN BETWEEN

Not only does the breath provide a way to sense into the different layers of the body and being, the still points hidden within its movement emerge as little doorways into the infinite. It's here where the yogi can place her/his single pointed focus for a taste of that seamless state of formless being which resonates as joy.

Expanding these still points became an essential focus in medieval yoga practices. Mallinson and Singleton (2017, p.131) explain that breath retention, *kumbhaka*, remains the 'ultimate breath practice' in many of the *haṭha* texts. They also mention that there is a preliminary practice called *sahita kumbhaka* where retention is accompanied by inhalation and exhalation (and that this type of *prāṇāyāma* differs considerably in expression and approach across the texts).

I prefer what I consider a 'soft' interpretation of this latter approach in the breath awareness practices of Restorative Yoga. In fact, I tend to not even think of retention at all, but rather a savouring or lingering in the stillness amid the breath's movement. It's here in this space in between that a tangible and felt sense of ecstasy can arise.

One of my favourite texts, the *Vijñāna Bhairava Tantra* (VBT), which was written in the 9th century before Tantra came to its zenith (11th–12th centuries) and well before *haṭhayoga* fully emerged as a complete system (15th century), describes a meditation practice that works with the current of the breath and points towards the still points in between the breath's movement as a means to experience inner fullness (Lakshman Joo 2007).[3] It has become the framework on which I base many of the breath awareness practices in Restorative Yoga (although it isn't the only way to work with the breath).

---

2   Senthilnathan, S. *et al.* (2018) 'An investigation on the influence of yogic methods on heart rate variability.' *Annals of Noninvasive Electrocardiology*, 24(1), e12584, www.ncbi.nlm.nih. gov/pmc/articles/PMC6931825. This study reveals the relationship between attention and breathing as a powerful combination which affects heart rate variability (HRV) and which may help yoga practitioners derive long-term physiological benefits.

3   *ūrdhve prāṇo hyadho jīvo visargātmā paroccaret utpatti-dvitaya-sthāne bharaṇād bharitā sthitiḥ* – The exhaling breath should ascend and the inhaling breath should descend, (both) forming a *visarga* (consisting of two points). Their state of fullness (is found) by fixing them in the two places of (their) origin.

Described in *śloka 24* of the VBT, the inhale (*jīva*) descends and the exhale (*prāṇa*) ascends.[4] I prefer this directionality of the breath as taught in the VBT as it works in tandem with the movement of the diaphragm in a manner that calms the physiology and promotes more efficient breathing.[5]

As the breath softly descends on the inhale, it can draw the energy of the thinking mind literally down into the feel of the body, supporting embodied presence; it also moves with the natural broadening and slight descent of the diaphragm so necessary for an efficient inhale. The exhale softly ascends as it flows upwards and outwards releasing bodily tension, and can be used as a means to gently elongate the spine. Both the inhale and exhale trace an inner pathway that heightens the feel of the subtle body where the central channel, *suṣumnā nāḍi*, can be sensed.

When following the flow of the breath, the still points of the breath become palpable. In her book, *Meditation for the Love of It*, Sally Kempton (2011, pp.95–96) describes the 'technical term for the still point between two phases of movement' as *madhya*. In Sanskrit, this word literally translates to mean 'central' or 'middle' (Grimes 1996, p.178), and it can refer to the still points between the breath.

There is an amusement park where I grew up in Amarillo, Texas, with a ride named 'The Rainbow' where you swing from side to side. There is a part of the ride where you drop down into a freefall which summons a hearty scream, arms raised up towards the sky. But when ascending to the top of the swing there is a moment where the ride hangs suspended in mid-air. The breath stops and there is a split second of pure stillness and no thought (there also happens to be the most stunning view of the sunset) that is exhilarating. To me, that's a '*madhya*' – a 'middle' moment of pure stillness where time stops and the joy of pure being flashes forth.

There is another word in Sanskrit that refers to the 'centre or core of something' (its 'middle' so to speak), and that is *hṛdaya*, which translates to mean 'essence' or 'heart'. It also refers to the place 'where breath is still in the state of

---

4   Understand that not only does *prāṇa* refer to the broad sense of energy pervading and animating the world, it also refers to the specific winds or *vāyus* in the body that oversee its functioning. Here, *prāṇa* refers to the exhale.

5   The way the breath moves in this context demonstrates the variation of approaches among the different schools of yoga as some schools teach the exact opposite. I long ago set aside judgement of what's right or wrong in yoga practice as it varies so widely. Rather, subjective experience becomes the measure for success.

merging' (Grimes 1996, p.138). In the 11th-century text, the *Pratyabhijñā-hṛ-daya*, written by the Kashmiri sage Kshemaraja, a disciple of Abhinavagupta, expanding the *madhya*, or centre, is a practice used to attain the bliss of consciousness (Shantananda 2003).

From these two Sanskrit words, which crossover in meaning, we can see how the spaces between the breath become an entryway into the transcendent heart or essence of being; how inhale-linger, exhale-linger becomes an effective focus for Restorative practice and for diving deep into embodied presence.

Breath flows softly in and down and merges into the inner heart or soul space and there's a lingering, a savouring. Breath flows upwards and outwards and merges with the wide and spacious sky of pure being. Inhale affirms the form – the felt sense of the body receiving the fullness of the breath. The exhale affirms the formless – the felt sense of the body softening into the state of pure being beyond form. Two places or 'spaces' of stillness hidden within the breath that teach what it feels like to be free of separating thoughts and tendencies, anchored in pure, resonant being.

Breath remains the perfect teacher. If we draw on the lens of the 'Tantrik Five-Layered Self', the breath feels and is felt through the movement of the body – a vibrant pulsation that tirelessly expands and retracts. Breath mirrors the thoughts and emotions of the psyche, while a conscious focus stabilizes and grounds the mind. Breath also provides a vital bridge that re-connects the body–mind through present moment awareness. *Prāṇa* flows through the breath as an enlivening force that animates and supports life. The source of the breath reveals stillness and space as its foundation. Awareness exists as the underlying power of pure being expressing itself through all these layers – an undivided source that is ever-present.

In this way, the Restorative postures offer an accessible means to become intimate with the breath and thus the inner world. As a subtle vehicle, the impulse and intelligence of the breath illumine the very centre of being. The breath not only adjusts the physiological state contributing to wellbeing, it provides an unerring inner pathway with regard to spiritual endeavour.

Let's now look at the anatomy and physiology of respiration to better understand the breath's functioning, in order to support its free movement.

Chapter 9

The Anatomy and Physiology of Respiration

BACKGROUND

Efficient breathing not only enhances health and wellbeing, it also reflects a physiology in balance. If we understand its anatomy and physiology, breath becomes a powerful tool with which to realize the purpose of Restorative practice – to experience a relaxed, grounded and centred state. Instruction and approach can align with nature's design.

To sustain life, each cell of the body requires a supply of oxygen. Within the amniotic fluid environment of the womb, oxygen comes from the mother's respiratory system. Within an outer environment of air which contains 78 per cent nitrogen, 21 per cent oxygen, and 1 per cent argon and other gases, our own independent respiratory system takes in oxygen through thoracic respiration and ventilation (commonly referred to as breathing) and through cellular respiration.

Having no long-term storage sites for oxygen, an adult breathes an average of 12–18 breaths per minute within a normal resting rate in order to support life. This constant and vital exchange of oxygen and carbon dioxide (which is the waste product of respiration) serves as an underlying rhythm of aliveness from which energy is sourced, and therefore deserves more attention and understanding.

HOW OXYGEN GETS TO OUR CELLS

While breathing through the mouth is possible, and indeed will happen if there is a high demand for oxygen, the nose is specifically and especially designed for breathing. It has raised prominences called conchae which act like turbines to circulate the air in its passages, preparing it for the gaseous exchange in the lungs. Their unique shape not only enhances filtering of the air by hairs (cilia) and mucous secretions, but capillaries close to the surface within the nose slightly warm the air on an inhale as it passes through the conchae and oral passages.

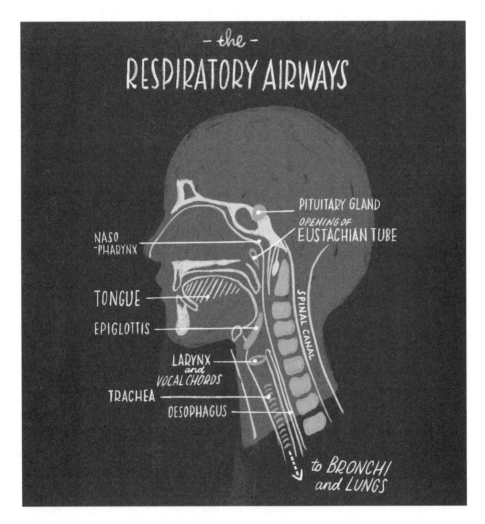

Air then enters the airway passages of the pharynx and then the larynx (where vocalization occurs via the 'vocal cords'). From here it enters the trachea, the ridged tube felt at the front of the throat formed of fibrocartilaginous rings.

The trachea rests in front of another tube, the oesophagus, which goes to the stomach. At the top of the trachea is the epiglottis, a curious and important little flap of fibrocartilage which covers the opening of the trachea when swallowing, to direct food and liquids to the stomach, rather than the lungs. When this flap doesn't work well, something can get 'stuck in our throat', resulting in a need to cough to clear the blockage.

From the trachea, the air then enters the bronchi and bronchioles in the lungs, ending up at the alveoli where the gaseous exchange of oxygen and carbon dioxide with the blood takes place. The alveoli are tiny air sacs clustered in bundles resembling a bunch of grapes; their round shape optimizes the surface area available for gaseous exchange to take place within the confined space of the thoracic cavity. If all of the alveoli were opened up (there are roughly 300 million of them within the lungs), they would cover an area equivalent to a tennis court! The alveoli have very thin cell walls, which facilitates the diffusion of oxygen and carbon dioxide molecules between the atmosphere and the blood, a delicate balance which directly impacts the body's functioning.

On crossing this thin cell wall, the oxygen molecules bind themselves to haemoglobin found in the red blood cells, which transports them around the circulatory system until they reach a cell in need. Released from the haemoglobin, oxygen enters the cell by diffusion.

It's interesting to note that anatomically the right and left lungs are different sizes. As the smaller of the two, the left lung consists of two lobes (or compartments), while the right lung consists of three. The reason for this is that the heart occupies a lot of space. Located between the right and left lungs in the mediastinum, it sits over to the left, reducing the space available for the left lung. As a result, the right lung on inhalation accounts for about 60 per cent of air intake, and the left lung about 40 per cent.

CELLULAR RESPIRATION AND THE PRODUCTION OF ENERGY (ATP)

When entering the cell, oxygen molecules along with glucose are used in the process of metabolism to produce adenosine triphosphate (ATP), which is the main energy currency of a cell. Most of this process occurs within a mitochondrion, an organelle inside the cell which generates most of the cell's supply of ATP. When energy is released with oxygen, it's called 'aerobic respiration'. When energy is released directly from glycogen (the storage form of glucose) without oxygen (a faster process), it's described as 'anaerobic respiration'.

One of the by-products of cellular respiration is carbon dioxide. As a waste product, it needs to be transported back to the lungs in order to be removed; this is done via the circulatory system either as bicarbonate (a compound of the gas carbon and water) dissolved in plasma or combined with protein substances in plasma. Through the gaseous exchange which occurs at the alveoli, carbon dioxide then enters the lungs and is released through an exhale.

THE ANATOMY AND PHYSIOLOGY OF THORACIC RESPIRATION

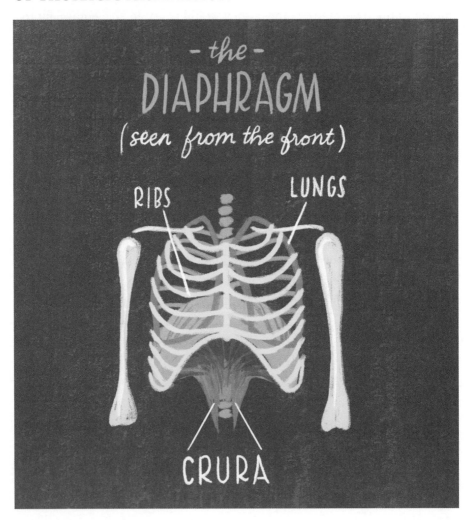

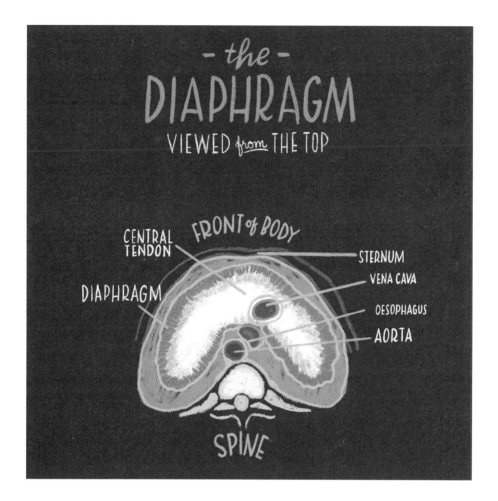

Inhalation

The diaphragm is the primary muscle of respiration accounting for about 70 per cent of the intake of air. The diaphragm contracts for inhalation to occur, having been stimulated by the phrenic nerve, whose nerve roots leave the cervical spine at the levels of C3, 4 and 5 ('C' referring to the cervical vertebrae of which there are seven). The contraction and very slight descent of the diaphragm increases the volume of the thorax. Following Boyle's law, this reduces the pressure in the lungs relative to the atmosphere such that air will be drawn in – a pressure gradient created with the atmosphere. (Boyle's law states that for a fixed amount of gas at a constant temperature the volume of gas is inversely proportional to the pressure of the gas. Therefore, as the volume of gas decreases the pressure will increase and vice versa.)

Origin
Back of the xiphoid process.

Lower six ribs and their costal cartilages.

Upper two to three lumbar vertebrae (L1–L3).

Insertion
All fibres converge and attach onto the central tendon.
(The diaphragm is the only muscle that inserts onto itself.)

Nerve supply
Phrenic nerve (C3, 4 and 5).
The accessory muscles of respiration, which assist the diaphragm on inhalation, are the external intercostals, the scalene muscles and sternocleidomastoid in the neck.

On inhalation, the lower nine ribs move out to the sides in a movement resembling lifting a bucket handle, while the top three ribs are raised in a pump handle action. Focusing on the natural movement of the ribs and diaphragm, while allowing the neck muscles and shoulders to quieten, supports an efficient inhale.

Exhalation
Exhalation is a passive process – the diaphragm relaxes and the lungs have elastic recoil. This reduces the volume of the thorax and, again following Boyle's law, the pressure within the lungs relative to the atmosphere is increased. To balance the pressure gradient that is created, air moves from the lungs back out to the atmosphere. The abdominal muscles of rectus abdominus, the internal and external obliques and transversus abdominus can be recruited in 'forced expiration'. Moving with the natural release of the diaphragm, lungs and ribs supports an efficient exhale.

For both inhale and exhale, an efficient breath initiates through the diaphragmatic and rib movement and is actuated through the pressure gradient as explained by Boyle's law; in this sense, there is no need to grasp for or push out the breath.

STRESS AND THE RESPIRATORY SYSTEM

While there is a degree of voluntary control over the respiratory system (the ability to consciously take a deeper breath), it is fundamentally under the control of the autonomic nervous system, which is strongly influenced by the mechanisms of the stress response. With stimulation of the sympathetic nervous system and adrenalin, both the rate and depth of respiration are increased. Furthermore, the bronchi dilate to increase the intake of oxygen for fight or flight. The increase in the rate and depth of heart beat ensures an increased delivery of oxygen (and glucose) to the cells for metabolism and the production of energy.

It is not surprising that the effects of long-term stress can become apparent within the respiratory apparatus. This may manifest as short, rapid, panicky breaths using only the upper part of the lungs, and chronic tension held in the neck and throat through the recruitment of the scalenes, sternocleidomastoid and subclavius. One can expect a tightening of the pre-cervical and pre-tracheal fascia along with the diaphragm, all of which cue the nervous system towards a sympathetic chain. Inevitably, this results in posture where the front of the body folds forward and contracts, restricting the full and efficient function of the respiratory system. When long term, these effects can be debilitating; by using knowledge of the anatomy and physiology of breathing, they can be countered.

Because the sympathetic nervous system is slightly stimulated on the inhalation, and the parasympathetic nervous system on the exhalation, lengthening the exhalation offers one of the easiest ways to counter the effects of the stress response and encourage the system to return to homeostasis. Aerobic exercise generally enhances respiratory function as long as performed regularly, moderately and enjoyably. Conscious relaxation can help release tension which interferes with breathing. From the perspective of structural shape and movement, exercises and postures which encourage chest opening (like back arches) and which facilitate freedom of movement within the spine and the ribs (like twists and forward folds) mean that you can literally take a deeper breath.

Chapter 10

———

A Free and Easeful Breath

A TRANSFORMATIVE AGENT

A free and easeful breath remains at the heart of Restorative practice; discovering what this means could be considered its art. Having explored the breath as teacher and friend and reviewed its anatomy and physiology, let's reflect on how best to free it, promoting the state of connection and ease.

Habitual movements, poor posture and prolonged stress form patterns of holding that disturb the breath's natural expression. By interfering with the free movement of the diaphragm, which directly influences state, these patterns become embedded changing the frame through which reality is perceived and experienced. Aptly expressed by Alexander Muacevic and John R. Adler in the conclusions to their 2018 study on the function of the diaphragm, 'Breath is a behavior. Behavior represents the person. Breath reveals the person.' Restricted by tension, the diaphragm's inability to work properly and descend on the inhale conveys danger or threat, triggering a low-grade sympathetic response (Rosenberg 2017).

The ability to see or sense patterns of holding and initiate a process of release through a free and easeful breath constitutes a significant part of Restorative practice as a transformative agent. The breath's expression offers a tangible way to feel how and where deep-seated tension is held; the power contained within its soft flow helps to release embedded patterns, supporting a profound shift of state.

A Restorative practice or class helps to release physical tension and encourages connecting with a more conscious, free and easeful breath, both powerful tools in bringing about a relaxed, grounded and centred state.

———

TENSION AS REVEALER

I often say in classes to follow the pulsation of the breath as a way to sense patterns of holding not only in the body, but within the breath itself. Along with time spent in postures, the breath's unfolding touch and rhythm reveals (and begins to transform) chronic patterns of holding which render the body opaque to nuance and depth. Attending to the breath's expression can ease these patterns and shift the physiology towards 'rest and digest', particularly when attention is placed on the exhale.

While tension in and of itself isn't bad (sometimes it's what's needed to expand), it is the chronic 'below the radar' kind restricting the breath which flattens experience. Learning how to release unnecessary tension recognizes the two-way communication between the body and mind where anxious holding patterns feed back to the central nervous system, reinforcing tones of fight or flight; where the release of tension in the diaphragm promotes restitution, social engagement and the experience of fullness of being.

To practise and eventually teach Restorative Yoga involves understanding and respecting tension for what it reveals. Learning how to release tension that interferes with the free movement of the diaphragm involves a gradual process of recognition and re-patterning. The ability to notice when, where and how tension hampers the breath's expression offers a skillset and pathway to an experience of freedom.

BECOMING AWARE

Awareness is the first step in releasing unnecessary tension and freeing the breath. The timeframe of practice allows space for held tension (whether physical or emotional) to rise to the surface enabling a process of recognition and release. Once a pattern is known, therein lies its attenuation. The Restorative approach asks for patience, presence and a willingness to stay with a process that results in the experience of softening and opening. But sometimes there can be choppy waters, where becoming still feels like the very last thing to do. And that's because 'doing' doesn't fit the process of release. Only 'being' does.

The Restorative ethos engenders gentleness, kindness and self-compassion, where there is permission and space to gently sense into and accept patterns of holding that limit the breath's expression. Allowing what is present to be there recognizes holding patterns as a type of survival mechanism. By embracing a pattern for what it is – a form of protection that's turned into a chronic limitation

– the energy caught up in tension, resistance and avoidance can gradually be released and redirected towards rest and recuperation.

Awareness serves as a healing balm that embodies the state of integration; gravity becomes a navigating force for the release of tension. To rest involves feeling safe enough to allow the power of Earth herself to rise up and extend the nurturing embrace of a mother. When held in this embrace, the power of yield dissolves tension and allows movement towards connection. The body speaks to the Earth and, in return, she teaches the interrelationship between body, breath, gravity and release.

As unnecessary tension dissolves, the breath can be felt and followed as a means of awakening to the richness of human experience. 'Feeling, sensing, noticing, experiencing' become descriptive means for subjective experience, where awareness shifts the paradigm of 'doing' into one of 'being'.

RELEASING TENSION THROUGH STRETCHES

Conscious and mindful stretching combined with breath awareness supports the depth of Restorative practice. Stretches help raise awareness of restrictive patterns of holding, and offer a simple means to release tension. Stretches also bring fresh blood to tissues constricted by tension, supporting healing and the movement towards balance. Not only do gentle stretches at the beginning of a sequence help to release tension, they also facilitate a free and easeful breath. Combined with the power of the breath's natural expression, stretches can help soften and integrate patterns of holding.

When releasing tension through stretches, the quality of stretching should be slow, deliberate and breath-initiated to avoid activating a sympathetic response. Moving consciously and slowly, particularly through the spine, warms up the body, focuses the mind and establishes the felt sense as arbiter in the release of tension.

The inhale can be used as a way to feel and sense into what is present, and the exhale as a way to soften and deepen a stretch within a range that is appropriate. If the breath suspends, come back from the depth of a stretch until the breath evens out, allowing for presence and awareness.

The following movements can be incorporated as gentle stretches (usually towards the beginning of a Restorative sequence) to help release tension and free the breath:

- *Hip stretches* – stretching the hips in all directions can help release a dynamic of tension within the pelvis and lumbar region that can impact the free movement of the diaphragm, which attaches to the lumbar spine.

- *Rotation* – rotating the spine stretches and releases tension in the muscles of the torso, creating more space for the ribs and lungs to move with the breath; it also stretches and releases tension in the diaphragm, encouraging a natural, deeper and fuller breath.

- *Lateral stretches* – stretching/contracting the side or lateral body supports the bucket-handle movement of the ribs which works in concert with the slight descent and contraction of the diaphragm. It also releases tension along the spine, which facilitates an easeful structure and diaphragmatic movement.

- *Gentle spinal extension/flexion* – extending the spine creates more space in the front body for the heart and lungs and counteracts the common tendency of collapsing the chest which restricts breathing; it also strengthens the muscles of the back which support healthy posture, and releases unnecessary tension in the upper body. Flexing the spine opens up the back of the body, allowing for a deeper breath into the lungs, which extend all the way down to the tenth rib at the back of the body. It also releases tension at the back of the neck/skull.

  Stretches help prepare the body for the deep rest of the Restorative poses, where the body can move with the tidal pulsation of the breath. When the body is softly receptive, the exhale can empty out unnecessary tension; the inhale can take in vital nourishment – a natural exchange from inside to outside and back again, where emptiness and fullness reflect the power of embodied presence. The responsive body serves as a sacred vessel for the experience of essence touched on so beautifully in this verse from the *Haṭhapradīpikā* compiled by Swātmārāma and translated by Akers (2002, p.98), 'Empty within, empty without, empty like a pot in space. Full within, full without, full like a pot in the ocean.'[1]

---

1 Most translations render *śūnya* as void rather than 'empty' as it is translated here. I prefer this poetic translation by Akers, as it conveys the quality of space as both empty and full.

COMMON AREAS OF HOLDING

During Restorative practice, there are common areas where tension hides. Interestingly, but not surprisingly, most of these areas are near the pathway of the vagus nerve and the other cranial nerves that comprise the parasympathetic nervous system (PSNS). These areas can be addressed through awareness and alignment to help release patterns of holding that support nervous system health and encourage a free and easeful breath.

- *The base of the skull* – offers one of the most powerful places to effect a global release of tension in the body. By adjusting the base of the skull at the back gently upwards, and softening the skin of the face downwards, a defensive pattern of tension ingrained as a baby through the 'Moro reflex'[2] can be eased. Eyes, face and jaw can soften, which supports the state of social engagement and connection. The adjustment of the back of the skull upwards also moves the hyoid bone up and back, releasing the root of the tongue, which attaches to it. This action domes the soft palate, creating a sense of space in the skull, throat and neck, as well as releasing tension in the face and abdomen.[3]

    This small but profound adjustment also counters the negative effects of 'forward head' where the position of the head pulls the weight of the skull down and forward on the atlas, loading the smaller sub-occipital muscles and the upper trapezius and sternocleidomastoid (all involved with positioning the head and fine tuning perception) with chronic tension. Forward head contributes to the collapse of the upper body, which restricts breath capacity by limiting space for the lungs and heart, as well as the ability to lift the first rib during inhalation (Rosenberg 2017). Simultaneously adjusting the sides of the neck back, and the base of the skull upwards, releases tension in these muscles usually recruited for alertness and defence, promotes healthy alignment necessary for breathing with ease and facilitates blood flow to the brain, supporting the health of the cranial nerves which oversee the parasympathetic response.

---

2   Christopher W. Edwards and Yasir Al Khalili (2020) describe the Moro reflex (which is sometimes called the startle reflex) as an involuntary movement a baby makes when startled – extending the arms and opening the hands accompanied by a slight throwing the head back followed by drawing the hands to the front before releasing the arms down: https://www.ncbi.nlm.nih.gov/books/NBK542173.

3   Richard Rosen likens this adjustment to an opening of the third eye – that place in the subtle anatomy where consciousness begins its upward ascent into the higher realms of being.

- *The neck and shoulders* – when placed with awareness this creates tangible space and softness through the neck, which supports calming. Combined with the skull adjustment, moving the shoulders gently back and softening the shoulder blades down away from the ears supports the release of tension in the upper trapezius, neck muscles and face. The expression, 'C3, 4, 5 keeps the diaphragm alive' refers to the phrenic nerve, which originates in the neck or cervical spine – it provides motor and sensory input to the diaphragm. By keeping the back of the neck long there is space to support the optimal functioning of this vital and important neural pathway for breathing.

  Always check the neck/skull alignment in the Restorative postures, so that there is softness and length in the neck, and space at the base of the skull. In the supine position, adjust the forehead so that it is slightly higher than the line of the chin. Fully support the head and neck with the right height of blankets to allow softening and to rest the back. This releases unnecessary tension in a key area where autonomic state is regulated and where ideal alignment supports the conditions for softness, free breathing and a sense of wellbeing.

  Simple, gentle neck stretches before doing the Restorative postures or even during a sequence can go a long way towards releasing tension in this area, supporting a parasympathetic response.

- *The face and eyes* – have much to do with regulating state. In *The Pocket Guide to the Polyvagal Theory*, Stephen Porges (2017) explains how facial expression has evolved to convey mutual safety and trust in such a way that can calm and downregulate defence. Eyes wide open indicates sympathetic activation, which prepares the body for fight or flight. Often this is reflected in fearful, tense body language. Focus on releasing tension in the face, especially the skin of the forehead, encouraging spaciousness between the eyebrows. Allow the eyes to soften back into the skull, releasing the upper eyelid and softening the gaze. Generally, the eyes are closed in Restorative Yoga to facilitate a quieting of the nervous system, as well as an inward focus. Note: if someone feels uncomfortable with closing the eyes, then simply encourage them to soften the gaze and release the upper eyelid to about halfway. It's more important for them to feel safe and at ease to support the shift of the physiology.

- *The tongue* – when tensed this creates hardness in the throat and diaphragm. Releasing the tongue softens the throat and solar plexus, facilitating the free movement of the diaphragm and fullness in breathing. Releasing the root of the tongue opens the back of the throat, promoting an internal softness which may positively impact the functioning of PSNS cranial nerves, innervating the tongue, upper throat and face. Compelling points raised by Rosenberg (2017) on the function of the cranial nerves and regulating state seem to correlate with yoga alignment and work nicely in the context of Restorative practice. Softening the tongue also seems to help the mind settle. A non-verbal mode of being supports an inward subjective experience; subtle realms can be explored through the felt sense without the effort of having to describe or explain.

- *The solar plexus, diaphragm and abdomen* – when gripped, this restricts the movement of the respiratory diaphragm and the ability to breath with ease. Holding in this area can arise from clothes that are too tight or unconscious tensing brought about by fear. Consciously releasing the solar plexus and abdomen allows space for the diaphragm to move freely. Placing the hands on the solar plexus helps to bring awareness to this part of the body, encouraging softening and the release of tension. Again, releasing the tongue encourages a softening. Sensing the movements of the diaphragm through the hands – a soft circular expansion on the inhale, a gentle release and condensing on the exhale – helps cultivate a healthy breath pattern.

- 'The three diaphragms'– pelvic, respiratory and thoracic diaphragms, when misaligned, can result in unnecessary tension and strain. I first came across 'the three diaphragms' as a concept through the insightful and subtle work of Donald Moyer in his book, *Yoga: Awakening the Inner Body* (2006, p.63). He suggests envisioning the three diaphragms as 'flat, circular planes passing through the circumference of each diaphragm to develop awareness of the horizontal planes of the body'. Sensing the alignment and tonality of the diaphragms, both individually and in relationship to each other, creates space through the spine, releases tension and subtly adjusts the flow of the breath. Aligning the centre of the diaphragms/circles along a vertical axis, and then adjusting the front, side or back edges of the circles of the diaphragms according to what is needed in a pose, results in a deep internal softening and settling of the bony structure that allows for integration and a free and easeful breath.

Creating an environment of easefulness and safety, where people may begin to explore common areas of holding, forms a key part of the Restorative ethos. By releasing physical and mental tension through awareness and alignment, there is space to discover a free and easeful breath which supports balance and a centred and grounded state.

FOLLOW THE CURRENT OF THE BREATH

It's helpful to imagine the breath as like a current or a wave. It conveys a softness and fluidity that is multi-directional and adaptive, yet powerful. When the breath is felt and followed from this fluid stance, time dissolves within an infinite ebb and flow as breath circles through the body and back again. When tension interferes with this current, its flow becomes weakened and disturbed. As tension dissolves, the body becomes receptive to the breath's full flowing power, which rejuvenates and enlivens, opening the door to subtle experience.

Following the breath's current recognizes its innate intelligence. You don't have to do the breath. Rather, it does you. The unfettered breath expresses a natural rhythm and flow that becomes a means for diving deep inside to source joy. Restorative practice offers space to explore and discover what it feels like to experience a breath that has been freed. In this respect, it's helpful to contemplate the quality of a free and easeful breath, and consider what supports or interferes with its expression. Different words help illuminate and describe a free and easeful breath – how it feels in the body, and what it does:

- *Uninterrupted* – effortless and easeful with no striving or pushing, reflecting a natural rhythm that enlivens and supports.

- *Pulsates* – moves with the diaphragmatic impulse initiating from the centre of the torso; each cell within the body pulses with the breath.

- *Even and steady* – an even and steady breath arises from a calm backdrop and gifts presence.

- *Changeable* – responds to outer situations supporting what is needed in the moment, and then returns to evenness.

- *'Non-doing'* – a sense of 'being breathed', rather than 'doing' the breath.

- *Quiet* – non-grasping and unlaboured.

- *Paradoxical* – expresses multi-directional movement, as well as stillness within its full expression.

- *Longer exhale* – indicates being at ease and safe.

- *Seamless and fluid* – reflects a wholeness that flows through a responsive body.

- *Energetic* – *prāṇa*, the life force, flows through the medium of the breath, drawing forth vitality.

- *Flows* – from outside to inside and back again, like waves in the sea.

Inevitably, over the course of a lifetime, there will be times when the pattern of breathing becomes disturbed – the current of the breath impacted by the circumstances of life. During these times, Restorative practice helps re-establish the steadiness of a free and easeful breath. It offers space to witness and 'presence' the intensity of life's curveballs written in tension. Learning to sense these patterns, and effect change through awareness and breath, allows process and release.

I always come back to verse 24 of the *Vijñāna Bhairava Tantra* (Lakshman Joo 2007) to restore the natural movement of the breath, and to become aware of stillness. To feel the breath flow in and downwards, like a wave coming into shore, affirms the solidity of the body and the diaphragm's descent... To feel the breath flow upwards and outwards, like a wave that flows back out to sea, ascends the spine mirrored by the diaphragm's release. Every movement of the breath reveals stillness as its source – a tiny but mighty gap at the depth of the inhale and at the end of the exhale, where the mind can rest, even if only for a split second.

The diaphragm leads the breath's dance, its rhythm determined by the moment and what's needed. Through its movement, the body becomes a softness, a receptivity that allows a natural exchange where the power within the breath can nourish and cleanse – an ever-present solace revealing the power within.

Paying attention to the breath in this way expresses open listening. Breath serves as the primary way to adjust the physical body and the nervous system. By accenting the breath's natural expression, an engaged and intentional process empowers and softens. It allows an approach that offers subtlety of perception and, ultimately, transformation.

Chapter 11

―――――

Exploration and Enquiries

Drawing on the power of embodied presence and the breath as a teacher and friend, these enquiries help raise awareness around patterns of holding, encouraging a gradual softening that supports a free and easeful breath.

Any variation of *śavāsana* or *supta sukhāsana* (See Chapter 13, The Six Main Restorative *Āsana* and Variations) serves as a comfortable pose for exploration and enquiry. Pick a posture and settle into it. Adjust the shoulder blades down the back and smooth the skin at the back of the pelvis down. Adjust the base of the skull upwards and make sure there is enough support underneath the head, so that the forehead sits slightly higher than the chin. (All four enquiries can be adapted for meditation.)

Have a journal and pen ready.

FEEL AND FOLLOW YOUR BREATH

Begin to sense the breath's movements. What aspect of your breath do you notice first? What draws your attention? Be careful to allow the breath pattern that is present, rather than trying to 'fix' it. Stay with what you notice for a few rounds of breath. As you do, inevitably, the breath pattern will soften and deepen. Be sure to pay particular attention at the beginning.

Follow the pathway of the breath as it moves and notice how the body responds to its movement. If you observe/experience a pattern of holding, allow it to be there. Explore the feel, texture or dynamic of the pattern as the breath moves. Is it at the level of the physical body? Is it within the breath's rhythm? Is it a tensional pattern within the mind? What is the interrelationship? Be curious and gentle.

What words, images or sensations arise as you stay with your experience?

Now place the warmth of your hands on the solar plexus. Feel the breath's movement. Send the soft, healing energy of an inhale to that place which is holding. Draw on the releasing power of an exhale to gradually soften. Breathe in this way for a little while.

When you are ready, very gently, roll to the side and come up to sitting. Write about your experience in your journal.

EXPLORING THE LAYERS

Let's explore the layers of the body and being through the lens of the 'Tantrik Five-Layered Self'. (See Chapter 7, Embodied Presence, for a more detailed description of this roadmap for exploring conscious human embodiment.)

Allow the body to rest back into the support of the props, ground and gravity. Become aware of the way the body rests, sensing its shape and feel. What do you notice? Are there obvious tensional patterns? Is there sensitivity? Restlessness? Ease? Sense into the different parts of the body taking the support of the breath's pulsation as a way to feel. Notice what is present in the physical form, without judgement. Stay here for a little while.

Now feel into the layer of the psyche – the mental and emotional layer interwoven with body and breath. What is the tenor of the mind? What is the emotional state? Again, without judgement or going into the narrative of the mental and emotional story itself, experience the feeling of this layer. Where in the body do you feel it? How does it impact the breath's flow? Stay with this focus for a little while and see what arises.

Shift your attention now to the breath itself. Feel the vital energy or *prāṇa* within the breath – the enlivening force that sustains life. Sense its revitalizing power flowing in the feet…the legs…the torso…the arms and hands…the neck and head. (Take time in each place to feel into and sense aliveness.)

Now, widen perception and experience the body as an energetic whole, pulsing with *prāṇa*, the life's breath. Allow perception to shift into being breathed – a breath that is free and at ease. Feel the vitality of the breath extending beyond the body – the breath flows from outside to inside, and back again.

As the breath moves, notice the still points in between the breath's movement without actually stopping the breath. Feel into the underlying stillness from which the breath arises and subsides…empty of the form of things, transcendent with the fullness of being. Rest in the awareness of these still points for a while.

Now lean into the very core of this stillness, and sense consciousness or awareness – touch that part that knows that it knows. Allow the joy of pure being to arise – the power of presence interpenetrating all the layers. Presence as centre…as stillness…as breath…as mind…as body… Joy flowing forth from the centre.

Place the hand on the solar plexus and take two or three deep breaths. Roll onto your side and come up to sitting. Sit quietly for a short while. Then write about your experience in your journal.

BIRD'S WINGS

Drape the hands across the front ribs – thumbs and index finger on the ribs; middle, fourth and little fingers across the solar plexus. Make sure the elbows are supported and relax the shoulders.

Feel the movement of the diaphragm through the touch of the hands, and internally. On the inhale, experience the soft expansion of ribs and diaphragm like a bird's wings opening outwards to soar. On the exhale, their gentle release is like a bird landing on a branch, folding her wings in to rest. Stay with this image for a little while, exploring the breath's movement without forcing.

Now place the fingers at the side ribs in a way that is comfortable. Feel the sideways movement of the ribs, opening outwards on the inhale…releasing on the exhale. This movement is often described as a 'bucket-handle' movement. Breathe into the hands lifting the handle of the bucket outwards…and breathe out releasing the bucket handle back down again.

Rest the arms by the sides a little away from the torso. Bring the attention to the back ribs resting on the prop or ground. Breathe into the bottom tip of the lungs at the back, sending the breath softly downwards. Make the exhale long, releasing the back body more deeply into the support of gravity. Stay with this breath pattern for a while. Breathe back and down. Exhale and soften.

Now combine all three aspects. Allow the inhale to gently expand outwards, to the sides and back, and the exhale to softly release the body into the earth. Imagine the inhale as like a bird soaring in wide and spacious skies, and the exhale, a landing onto the earth's steady ground.

Gently reach the arms over the head and stretch through the whole body. Bend the knees and roll onto your side, and slowly come up to sitting. Write about your experience in your journal.

BREATH AS TEACHER AND FRIEND

Place your hands on the area of the solar plexus. Become absorbed in the movement of the diaphragm. As the inhale softly flows downwards from the nose into the lungs towards the hands, feel the supple expansion of breath, muscle and bone. As the exhale flows upwards and outwards, feel how the breath can elongate the spine and release the body more deeply into the earth. Stay with this current of the breath: the inhale flows downwards towards the hands and mirrors the expansion of the diaphragm; the exhale flows upwards and moves with the direction of the diaphragm's release.

There is a flow to the breath. And there is also an ebb. A fleeting still point at the depth of the inhale, and at the end of the exhale, so small that it's almost not there. See if you can touch the still point with your awareness without stopping the breath's flow.

What happens if you linger there for a short while, at that still point to either side of the breath's movement?

What happens to the mind in that split second of stillness? It's as if the mind stops – a profound and timeless pause hidden within the space between, like a pearl.

Begin to savour and cherish these still points.

After a while, allow the feel and texture of stillness to expand within like a balm to the soul. Without actually stopping the breath, these fleeting still points become an underlying, ever-present layer of spacious presence where the mind can rest. Where the body can rest. Where the being comes alive through the dance of the breath.

Let the breath become your teacher and friend.

Gently move fingers and toes. When ready, softly stretch through the whole body. Bend the knees and roll onto your side, and slowly come up to sitting. Write about your experience in your journal.

SUMMARY OF PART II

Embodied presence refers to a type of enquiry that unlocks the power of present moment awareness through a deeply felt sense of body and being. It expresses a conscious movement towards essence through the layers of being, and recognizes innate wisdom. Taking the support of a breath that is felt and followed, patterns of holding can be released, allowing fullness of being where inner joy can be sourced. Restorative Yoga allows for a transformative process where presence and breath offer a pathway towards integration and wholeness.

Part III

―――

PRACTICE

To engage in a deliberately slow and spacious practice includes mindful stretches, supported postures, breath awareness and meditation, all of which draw forth the mantle of wellbeing.

Chapter 12

———

Wellspring

THE LIVED EXPERIENCE OF BALANCE

Regular practice enlivens and supports the ability to convey the depth and beauty of Restorative Yoga. It facilitates a grounded and steady state from which instruction can resonate with power and presence.

Exploring the various set-ups and props creates a foundation of experiential knowledge from which to innovate and learn how to adapt the postures. In this way, practice becomes a wellspring from which embodied knowledge flows forth, imbuing teaching with creativity, clarity and compassion.

Periodically stepping out of the role of teacher and *experiencing* a Restorative class illuminates the process of relaxation in a way that strengthens its teaching. Undergoing a curated and progressive quieting enables the understanding of what works and what doesn't – the ability to give the right cues at the right time in order to support subtle experience.

Restorative practice prioritizes taking time to pause, feel and listen inwards; it invites the lived experience of balance, a necessary ingredient for teaching Restorative Yoga.

A NEW (OLD) DEFINITION OF DISCIPLINE

Yoga encompasses countless teachings and practices which refine perception and transform state. Teachers of the tradition have passed on this knowledge from one generation to the next in a manner that exemplifies discipline as well as compassion. Teaching Restorative Yoga (and indeed any style of yoga) involves cultivating a more refined understanding of *discipline* as a virtue that transforms practice and gives rise to the wish to help others.

———

The word discipline developed a negative tone from about the 1500s onwards when it took on connotations of punishment. In modern times, it's sometimes used in a way to imply cracking the whip when it comes to yoga practice, which can often be a deterrent. But in the earlier history of this word, discipline had another more enlightened interpretation linked to the word disciple. Coming from the Latin for 'pupil', *discipulus* is formed from a lost compound, *discipere*, which means 'to grasp intellectually, analyse thoroughly'. Another Latin word, *disciplina* translates as 'instruction and training' (Barnhart 1988, p.282). Drawing from these etymological strands, discipline can be viewed as a steady and consistent process of deep investigation and learning, where self-application has everything to do with discovery and assimilation.

This elevates the discipline of practice to one of immersion in essence, and becomes a process of illumination that liberates – a refinement that embodies a genuine effort made through practice to learn about the connection between self, soul and world. Stephen Cope elucidates this in his book, *The Great Work of Your Life* (2012, p.16), 'All true *dharma* is a movement of the soul back to its Ground.' And so the discipline of practice can be seen as the means...

Practice becomes a wellspring that ignites a transformative experience and becomes a source for living in balance and teaching with passion. In times of fragmentation, it offers sanctuary, sowing the seeds of connection vital for transmitting the experience. The discipline of practice and teaching Restorative Yoga become an uplifting means to serve human beings flourishing by recognizing and prioritizing connection. (More on this in Chapter 15, The Art of Teaching Restorative Yoga.)

Consider the approach to your practice. Take a moment and reflect. What is the tenor of your practice? What is the purpose of your practice? Consider your teaching. What is the felt sense of your teaching? Does it arise from the inspiration of tapping into your inner being? Take some time to write your thoughts about your practice in your journal, an *ātmavicāra*-style enquiry. Then lie down on the floor, put your hands on your body and breathe. What are you learning from the feel, rhythm and flow of your breath? What is the quality and texture of this unfolding moment? How does the body meet the floor? Is there rigidity? Is there yield? What is present in the innermost space of your heart and being? Enquire within. Then ask the quintessential question: *Why do I practise yoga?* And listen inwards...

Invoke the power of discipline in your practice with this new (old) definition of the word.

Chapter 13

The Six Main Restorative *Āsana* and Variations

OVERVIEW

There are broadly six main Restorative *āsana*, or postures, that include a number of variations which can be organized according to their shape: *supta baddha koṇāsana, balāsana, adho/ūrdhva mukha jaṭhara parivartanāsana, setubhanda sarvāṅgāsana, vīparita karaṇī* and *śavāsana*. The most common poses are covered in this way of conceptualizing the Restorative body of work, and it provides an easy way to work with sequencing and begin to teach postures.

There are a few other Restorative poses that don't quite fit this categorization: side lying poses; hybrid poses that cross categories; and more active and stretch-oriented postures such as a supported dog pose. For more in-depth study of the range of the curriculum and how to approach crafting Restorative poses, it's best to attend a formal Restorative Yoga teacher training which can cover the different possibilities.

Remember that Restorative poses are always supported in some manner, held for longer periods to allow a shift of the physiology, and support the ability to turn inwards. When combined with stretches and well crafted within an intentional sequence, the poses present many creative possibilities for bringing about a relaxed, grounded and centred state of being.

Each of the Restorative postures may affect the physiological state and the body in different ways. A pose that works for one person may not work for another as age, past experience, medical conditions and predisposition influence experience. It's important to discover the right variation which encourages relaxation and rest, and which also facilitates the breath.

ASSESSING A POSE

When assessing a Restorative posture in term of its potential benefits and effects, it's useful to consider a number of things:

- *Musculoskeletal dynamics* – which muscles are being stretched/contracted and the particular action at certain joints.

- *Shape of a pose and physiology* – consider how a particular system may be affected by a certain shape of pose. For example, how compression or relaxation of a body area might affect the flow of blood (haemodynamics) or the breath pattern.

- *Individual uniqueness and preference* – different people will find different postures beneficial. For example, *vīparita karaṇī*, also known as legs up the wall pose, may be uncomfortable for those with tight hamstrings and need to be adapted, or it could aggravate sciatica, in which case it's better to find another inverted variation that doesn't do these things.

- *Comfort and the ability to feel safe* – this aspect highlights the importance of an environment conducive to relaxation, which includes language, tone of voice and facial expression. Consider how words, movement and body language impact and support the experience of stillness and rest. (More on this in Chapter 15, The Art of Teaching Restorative Yoga.)

SUITABILITY

While for many people the Restorative poses serve as potent means for adjusting state and diving deep into experience, there are some considerations that may affect whether or not to practise in this way. If there is a specific condition or injury that may affect the ability to practise, it's best to seek advice from a medical professional to determine whether this style is suitable based on the individual's unique circumstances. There are four conditions that I'd like to mention:

- *Pregnancy* – the Restorative approach can be very supportive during pregnancy. That said, there are some aspects that need care and consideration, which may preclude certain postures and the time spent in a posture. For this reason, I recommend attending a specific teacher training designed for pregnancy and Restorative Yoga in order to apply safe practice.

Briefly, never rest directly on the belly or compress the abdomen *in any way* – this affects downward facing poses and rotations. Lying flat on the back can also present difficulty in that the weight of the foetus itself may impact the flow of oxygenated blood. For this reason, it's best to be well propped up in supine poses and/or to rest on the side. Practice during this time should be addressed individually with awareness of the complications that can arise due to hormonal shifts which impact flexibility.

- *Recent surgery* – it is best to rest and avoid physical practices until the wound has healed. Make sure to take advice from a medical professional before practising. Never put full weight on an area of sensitivity and avoid over stretching.

- *Spinal conditions* – such as spondylolythesis, spondylosis, scoliosis, sciatica and disc prolapse require medical advice and individual attention.

- *Post-traumatic stress disorder (PTSD)* – much research and study has come about in the past few years that has shed light on this condition, validating the experience of those who suffer from it, as well as the importance of how to treat it. While Restorative practices can be very helpful, again I recommend taking a specific yoga teacher training that addresses trauma and fosters understanding with regard to the best way to offer support. Consent to touch is non-negotiable, and permission to adapt the practice or pause when needed is quite important. Choice is fundamental in navigating the very real challenges that may arise during a practice for someone managing this condition.

In summary, every person is unique. Be respectful. Listen and work with a person when determining suitability and making adjustments. In the end, comfort and communication determine the best pathway forward.

UNIVERSAL APPLICATIONS

There are some general things that can be done across the board with regard to the architecture, alignment and comfort of a Restorative posture, all of which facilitate relaxation:

- *Place a blanket on top of a sticky mat* – spreading this underneath the whole of the body ensures that there is a foundation of softness that offers warmth, yet remains firm. A blanket that extends beyond the mat is helpful in cushioning elbows and hands that may end up resting on a cold, hard floor.

- *Support as much of the body as possible* – respecting individual uniqueness. Any major joint or part of the body suspended against gravity will eventually be felt. Fully propping the body encourages the sense of gravity as support. It minimizes intensity or the sensation of extreme stretch which may be stimulating to the nervous system, and reinforces an internal softness which frees the breath. Even supporting small spaces such as the inward curve of the neck or the back of the hand can make a huge difference in the ability to relax. In addition, take time to find the right height of support which allows for ease and restfulness.

- *Pick a texture of prop that is comfortable* – they can vary widely! Swapping out a new 'hard and high' bolster for an accordion folded blanket that is lower and softer may make all the difference in being able to stay in a pose.

- *Ground the body* – putting weight in key places on the body helps to release structural tension. This can be done through sandbags, buckwheat bolsters, folded blankets or eye pillows. Explore the best place to weight the body in order to release tension and promote rest. Remember that comfort drives choice and placement of prop.

- *Make sure there are plenty of blankets* – covering the body with a blanket or two can provide a sense of comfort, warmth and protection.

- *Anchor the tail of the spine down and adjust upwards from the base of the skull* – so that there is a sense of space running through the whole of the spine. When a person is supine, the forehead should always be slightly higher than the line of the chin. Check that the shoulders are soft and the shoulder blades comfortably adjusted down the back, away from the neck.

HOW TO FOLD A BLANKET

While a seemingly innocuous aspect, the method of folding a blanket contributes significantly to a comfortable set-up and the ability to stay in a pose.

In addition, there are times when a bolster is too high or two together are too thick. Learning how to fold a blanket accordion style allows adaptability in the height and width of a foundation.

Furthermore, always place the smooth edge of the blanket into the body as it provides a clean edge with which to align; shake out any wrinkles that may become the proverbial 'pea underneath the mattress'.

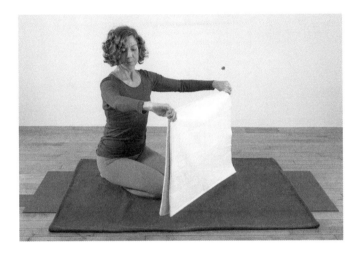

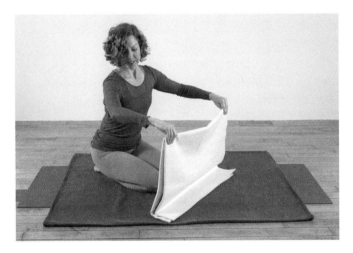

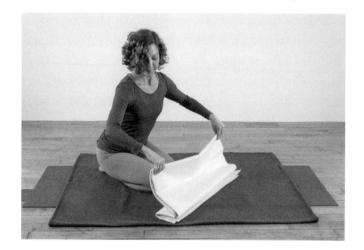

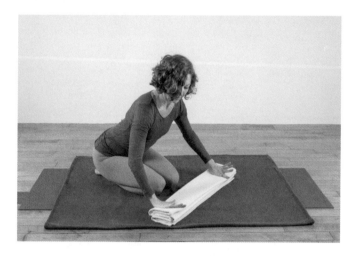

CONCLUDING REMARKS

I always get asked, 'How long do you hold a posture?' Of course the answer is, 'It depends.' A number of factors affect the time spent in a posture: where it's placed in a sequence, the unique situation of the person practising and the shape of the posture itself. Some poses have 'staying power' while others are brief interludes on the journey to *śavāsana*, which is, of course, the destination pose held for the longest period of time. (See Chapter 14, Sequencing.)

THE POSES
I. Supta baddha koṇāsana
Reclining Bound Angle Posture with a strap.

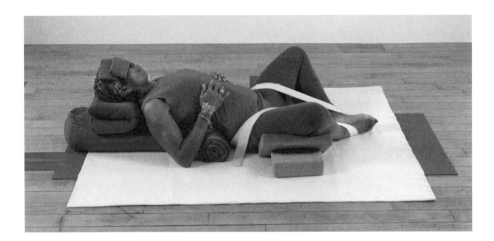

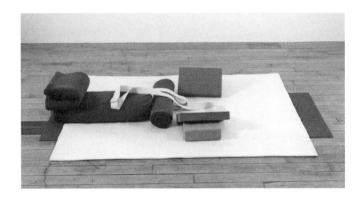

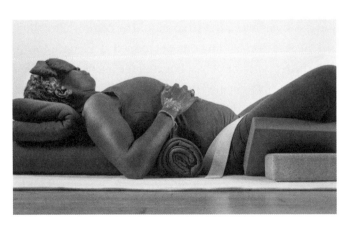

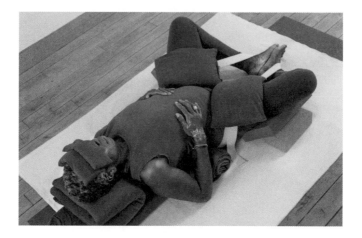

Props
Three blankets; one bolster; two foam blocks; two cork bricks; one strap; eye pillows and sandbags optional.

Timing
5–30 minutes.

Alignment awareness

- In order to encourage the torso to release into the bolster, place a rolled blanket at the bottom to extend a gradual descending support for the spine.

- Position the strap so that it is almost at the tailbone, ensuring it doesn't slide upwards into the lower back, which can cause compression. The strap's position at the tail anchors the spine, helping to maintain its length, especially in the lower back. The strap should be comfortably snug and secure to keep the feet from sliding out, yet looped at a length that allows space between the feet and the pelvis. Position the buckle free of the skin, and so that it can be easily tightened or loosened with the dominant hand. Always smooth the skin at the back of the pelvis down before and after placing the strap to maintain space in the lower back spine.

- Fully support the outer thigh and shin at an angle so that the hip creases remain soft and the knee joints are comfortable. Position the knees higher than the hips where there is no sense of strain or excessive stretch either at the knee, hip or inner thigh.

- Optional: place sandbags at the hip creases to anchor the thigh bones; slightly pull the sandbags towards the mid-line of the body to roll the thigh flesh inwards. Readjust the tailbone downwards towards the feet. Note: never place the sandbags on the knees.

- Pull the smooth edge of the blanket in to support the neck and head, not the shoulders; encourage the shoulders to roll back towards the bolster so the top of the chest is spacious and open. Position the forehead slightly higher than the line of the chin, creating space at the base of the skull.

- Optional: place one eye pillow across the brow. Then drape the second eye pillow across the first and over the bridge of the nose. This weights the forehead, releasing tension, and blocks out the light without putting weight on the eyeball itself. Note: eye pillows can be used throughout all the Restorative postures.

- Make sure the elbows, forearms and hands rest easily on the floor or on a prop so the arms and fingers are relaxed.

Anatomy and physiology

- Stretches the adductor muscles, gracilis and pectineus.

- Places the hips in external rotation with abduction.

- Creates space for the femoral vein, femoral artery and inguinal lymphatic nodes.

- Relieved of the downward pressure of gravity, allows space for the abdominal organs encouraging a freer flow of fluids (especially blood).

- Helps release myofascial tension in the pelvic floor, solar plexus, ribcage, shoulders and neck, which supports relaxation.

- Relaxes the diaphragm and supports easeful respiration.

- The support of the bolster gently extends the thoracic spine, opening the chest and creating more space for the lungs and heart, facilitating cardiac and respiratory function.

- Widens and spreads the clavicles, facilitating the opening of the thoracic inlet, which enhances lymphatic drainage back to the heart.

- Externally rotates the shoulders and lifts the sternum, supporting an optimal postural re-alignment.

- Relaxes pre-cervical fascia and muscles of the face, throat, neck and shoulders, aiding relaxation.

- Mildly stimulates the baroreflex via the baroreceptors in the carotid sinus in the neck, which has a quieting effect on the brain.

Considerations, cautions and contraindications

- Be cautious of knee or hip strains – consider raising the knees and adding more support under the legs and/or remove the strap and widen the distance between feet and pelvis.

- For discomfort in the lower back – swap out the bolster for accordion folded blankets 'stair stepped' to meet the curve of the back and adjusted to a comfortable height.

- For ankle strain, sprain or ligament problems – strategically place a thinly folded blanket underneath the feet/ankles for cushion and support.

- Some people may experience a feeling of vulnerability in this posture due to its open nature. Consider Variation 1 and cover the body with a blanket or ground it with a bolster to help provide a sense of comfort and protection. Consider Variation 2 as a less 'open' option.

VARIATION 1: *SUPTA BADDHA KONĀSANA*
Reclining Bound Angle Posture without a strap and with a bolster on top.

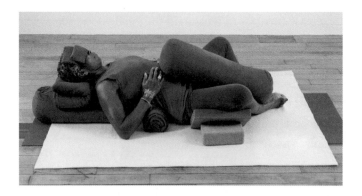

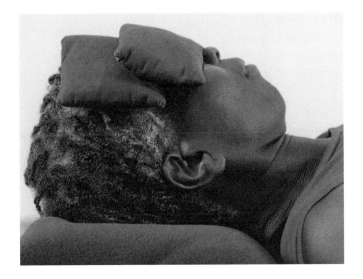

Props
Three blankets; two bolsters; two foam blocks; two cork bricks; eye pillow(s) optional.

Timing
Same.

Alignment awareness

- Same, minus strap instruction.

- Position the second bolster lengthwise on the front from the solar plexus to the feet – this helps keep the feet from sliding out. The bolster also helps to ground the body, assists with breath awareness and can address the sense of vulnerability that may arise when the abdomen is exposed.

Anatomy and physiology

- Same.

Considerations, cautions and contraindications

- Same.

VARIATION 2: *SUPTA SUKHĀSANA*
Reclining Easy Cross Legs Posture.

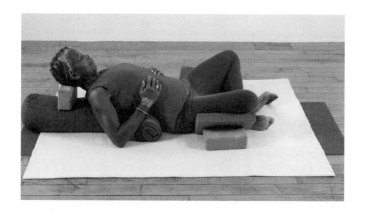

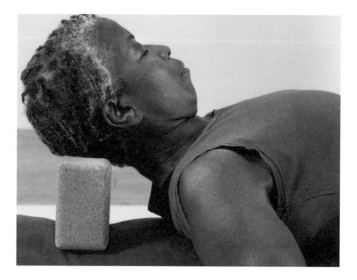

Props
Two blankets; one bolster; two foam blocks; three cork bricks.

Timing
Same – change cross of legs halfway through.

Alignment awareness

- Same, minus strap instruction.

- Cross the shins so the feet are in line with the knees; rest on the edges of the feet. Adjust the foam blocks in a way that supports the outer thigh, hip and knee comfort and the position of feet.

- Support the head with the middle side of the cork brick; place the edge of the brick at the base of the skull, so that the forehead is distinctly higher than the chin. Note: the edge of the brick should not be placed in the neck spine. If there is discomfort, place a thinly folded blanket across the top to add softness, or lower the brick, or simply swap out the brick entirely for a blanket.

Anatomy and physiology

- Same.

- The firmness of the brick can help to release muscular tension at the base of the skull and along the neck and upper back.

Considerations, cautions and contraindications

- Same.

- If the brick is too hard or there is irregularity with regard to the shape of the skull, place a thinly folded blanket across the brick or swap out the brick for a blanket. If there is strain along the back of the neck, lower the brick or use a blanket.

SUMMARY OF POSE AND VARIATIONS

The 'queen' of the Restorative postures, *supta baddha koṇāsana* and variations offer a calm, grounding and deeply restful pose that opens the front of the body and stretches the hips. It can be held for longer periods when fully supported. It is helpful for fatigue and menstruation due to its restful nature, and releases abdominal and pelvic floor tension through its position. Ideal for breath awareness practices at the beginning of a sequence.

II. Balāsana
Classic Child's Pose

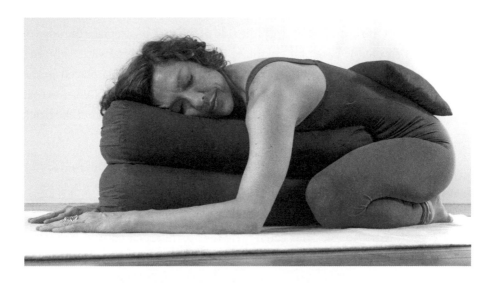

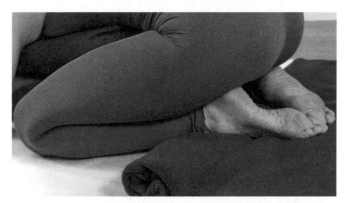

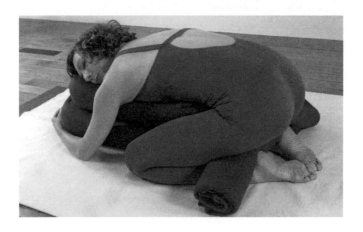

Props
One to three blankets; two 'flattish' bolsters; sandbag optional.

Timing
5–10 minutes – turn the head halfway through.

Alignment awareness

- The knees may require more cushioning in this posture. If so, place an additional blanket underneath the knees, shins and feet so the foundation is level and there is softness.

- When stacking the bolsters, pull the top bolster snugly in towards the pelvis so that the abdomen is fully supported. In this pose, the torso is parallel to the floor. Note: it may be that the bolsters are very large, in which case two will be too much. Lower the height by placing accordion folded blankets on top of one bolster to a height that suits.

- Hug the knees in around the bolsters so they touch it – if the knees are too wide it may overly stretch the inner hip joint in such a way that eventually results in pain or strain during a longer holding.

- Make sure the neck is soft and lengthened even when the head is turned to the side. Over the course of the posture, spend equal amounts of time with the head turned to each side. If there is discomfort when turning the head to the non-dominant side, come back to the original placement.

- Sit all the way back onto the heels – if the buttock bones do not reach the heels, roll a blanket and place it in between, so that there is support and grounding. This addition may require a higher lift for the torso, in which case add some accordion folded blankets on top.

- For people who may find putting weight through the ankle in this way uncomfortable, thinly roll a blanket and place it underneath the front of the ankle at the hinge to the width needed for ease in sitting back onto the feet.

- Optional: place a sandbag at the back of the pelvis towards the tail, to root the back and ground. Note: avoid this option if there is knee or ankle injury. This adjustment can be made across all variations of *balāsana* apart from Variation 1 – the raised torso makes the sandbag slide off.

Anatomy and physiology

- Stretches the front of the knees and ankles.

- Flexes hips and knees.

- Gently flexes the spine with forward folding shape of the body.

- Calms both physiologically and emotionally due to protected sense of the front body, which encourages feeling safe.

- Downward facing orientation tends to have a quieting effect – the passivity of the forward fold supports relaxation.

- Broadens the back body allowing for a deeper breath into the lungs (the lungs extend all the way to the tenth rib at the back of the body).

- Is restful for the heart as it doesn't have to pump blood up against gravity to the brain.

- Takes vertical weight off the spine lessening disc compression. Similarly, alleviates the downward compression of abdominal organs from gravity.

- Mildly stimulates the baroreflex via the baroreceptors in the carotid sinus in the neck, which has a quieting effect on the brain.

- Reduces lordosis of the lumbar spine, gently stretching the lower back muscles.

Considerations, cautions and contraindications

- For specific knee challenge, injury or conditions – place a rolled blanket or bolster in between buttock bones and heels, reducing the angle of knee flexion. If there is still pain, avoid this pose or, alternatively, practise Variation 6 of *adho mukha śavāsana* with legs stretched out.

- For hip discomfort, specific hip injury or conditions – use extra height under the torso to create more space at the hip joint, reducing the amount of hip flexion. If there is still pain, avoid this pose.

- For ankle restrictions or injuries – roll a blanket to the height needed and place underneath the front of the ankle. If there is still pain, avoid this pose.

- For restrictions in neck rotation, specified neck injuries or conditions – practise Variations 2 or 3 with head down to avoid rotating the neck.

VARIATION 1: *BALĀSANA*
Child's Pose with the torso lifted.

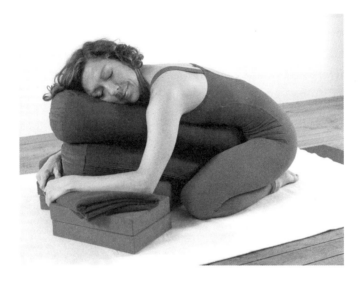

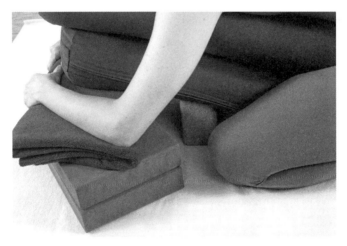

Props
One to three blankets; two 'flattish' bolsters; four foam blocks; one brick.

Timing
Same.

Alignment awareness

- Same, apart from the bolster placement which is more upright; make sure the brick underneath the bottom bolster lends support to the structure so it does not collapse. Ensure the lower abdomen is supported. Do not sit on the bottom bolster, rather rest back on the heels. Note: if the bolsters are firm, the cork brick may not be needed. If the bolsters are too high, swap out one for accordion folded blankets.

- Adjust the foam blocks so that the elbows and forearms are supported.

Anatomy and physiology

- Same.

Considerations, cautions and contraindications

- Same.

- Higher placement of the torso may increase pressure through the knees and/or ankle joints. Place a blanket accordingly. If there is still pain, avoid this pose or practise Variation 6 of *adho mukha śavāsana* with legs stretched out.

VARIATION 2: *BALĀSANA*

Child's Pose with the head down and bolsters placed lengthways with blanket across thighs.

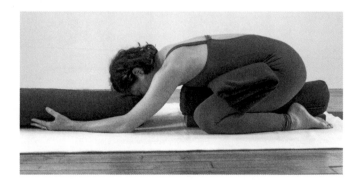

Props
One to three blankets; two bolsters; two foam blocks; sandbag optional.

Timing
5–10 minutes.

Alignment awareness

- Same, apart from bolster and blanket placement.

- When placing the bolster for the pelvis, raise it up on two foam blocks end to end. If needed, this can be made higher with more blocks or an accordion folded blanket to accommodate knee or ankle discomfort. More height eases the bend of the knees, hips and ankles.

- Sit towards the back of the bolster, so that the torso is fully supported when folding forward. Pull the smooth edge of a thinly accordion folded blanket placed widthways across the thighs deep into the hip crease. When coming forward into pose, tuck the front ribs slightly into the top edge of the blanket to spread the back ribs. The blanket helps release tension in the lower back. Make sure the fold of the blanket allows space for the chest. If there is discomfort, it's fine to remove the blanket.

- Optional: a sandbag drawn down towards the tail can be placed on the back of the pelvis to help ground the posture and keep the body from tipping too far forwards.

- When placing the bolster for the head, make sure the back of the neck is long and comfortable, and only the forehead rests on the bolster. The gap between the bolsters allows space for the face and breathing. If the bolster is too low, it may pull on the back of the neck; if the bolster is too high it may collapse the back of the neck. Adjust the height of the bolster accordingly using blocks or blankets. Cradle the hands around the bolster to create a widening across the shoulder girdle and a sense of release.

Anatomy and physiology

- Same.

- Releases tension at the back of the neck with forehead down, creating more space at the occipital base.

- Lengthens the ligamentum nuchae, which extends from the external occipital protuberance on the skull to the spinous process of C7.

- Helps to relax the facial muscles by resting the forehead on the bolster.

Considerations, cautions and contraindications

- Same.

- For abdominal discomfort, remove blanket.

VARIATION 3: *BALĀSANA*
Child's Pose with bolster placed widthways and blanket across thighs.

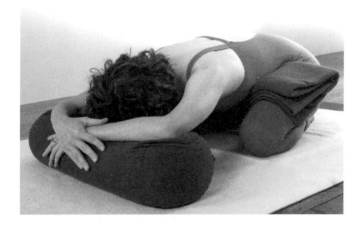

Props
One to three blankets; one bolster.

Timing
2–5 minutes.

Alignment awareness

- Same.

- Part the knees a little in line with the hips. Thinly accordion fold a blanket so that it acts like a sling for the belly and a support for the lower back. If there is abdominal discomfort, remove the blanket and proceed with a shorter holding.

- Position the bolster widthways so that the elbows and the forehead are supported and the sides of the body lengthened. When placing the forehead on the bolster, avoid pressing onto the nose, and softly lengthen up from the base of the skull, rolling towards the top of the forehead.

Anatomy and physiology

- Same.

Considerations, cautions and contraindications

- Same.

SUMMARY OF POSE AND VARIATIONS
This pose calms both physiologically and emotionally due to the protected sense of the front of the body, which encourages feeling safe. For many (not necessarily all) the forward folding position can comfort and nurture. It supports an inward focus and quieting of the mind through the downward placement of the head and supported forehead. It also quiets the senses of perception localized in the face and facilitates a back body breath and more efficient breathing.

III. *Adho mukha jaṭhara parivartanāsana*
Downward Facing Revolved Abdominal Posture with bent knees.

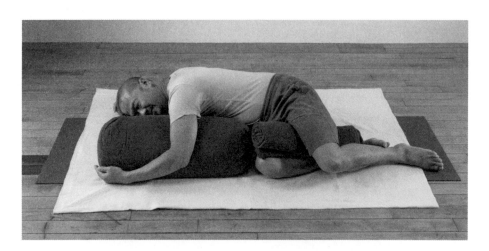

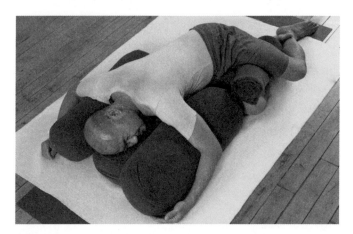

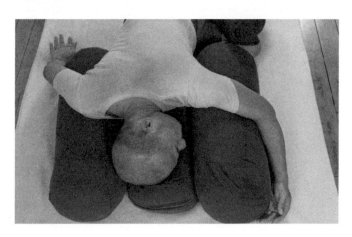

Props
Two blankets; three bolsters.

Timing
5–10 minutes, on each side.

Alignment awareness

- Place the middle bolster lengthways on the mat and centre the outer hip in line with the middle of the bolster; slightly angle the two outer bolsters upwards onto the middle bolster, so that the front of the shoulders are supported when lying over them. Spend time turning the abdomen so that the navel aligns with the middle of the bolster. Rest as much of the abdomen as possible downward facing on the bolster. Adjust the grounded hip away from the bottom of the bolster, so that the side waist stays long.

- Put a rolled blanket in between the thighs to prevent compression at the inner hip joints and to take pressure off the sacroiliac joints. This can be widened to relieve any sacroiliac discomfort.

- Place the arms so that the shoulders are supported at the front on the bolsters, and the hands cradle the bolsters. Note: for shoulder discomfort try folding one arm back in the direction of the rotation.

- Turn the head to the side that feels the most comfortable (usually the direction the knees are pointing). Adjust up from the base of the skull, ensuring that the neck feels spacious and long.

Anatomy and physiology

- Gentle rotation of the spine releases tension through a combination of contraction and relaxation of the abdominal corset muscles (obliques, transversus abdominus, quadratus lumborum and lower intercostal muscles), which also supports breathing.

- Stretches and releases tension in the diaphragm, encouraging a natural, deeper and fuller breath.

- Encourages perfusion, fresh blood flow, to the muscles of the back and abdominal organs.

- Supports peristalsis and digestive function.

- Takes vertical weight off the spine, lessening disc compression.

- Alleviates the downward compression of abdominal organs from gravity.

- Is restful for the heart as it doesn't have to pump blood up against gravity to the brain.

- Mildly stimulates the baroreflex via the baroreceptors in the carotid sinus in the neck, which will have a quieting effect on the brain.

- Downward facing orientation tends to have a more quieting effect.

- Encourages a feeling of safety due to the protected sense of the front of the body in downward facing arrangement.

- Broadens the back body allowing for a deeper breath into the lungs (the lungs extend all the way to the tenth rib at the back of the body).

Considerations, cautions and contraindications

- For lower back or sacroiliac challenges – proceed with caution. Place a wider support between the thighs. If discomfort continues, avoid asymmetrical postures and rotation.

- For neck discomfort – turn the head to the most comfortable side (which is usually the direction the knees are pointing) or practise the upward-facing Variations 2 or 3.

- For shoulder discomfort – place one or both arms downwards by the sides of the torso and ensure that the front of the shoulders is supported.

VARIATION 1: *ADHO MUKHA JAṬHARA PARIVARTANĀSANA*
Downward Facing Revolved Abdominal Posture with one leg straight.

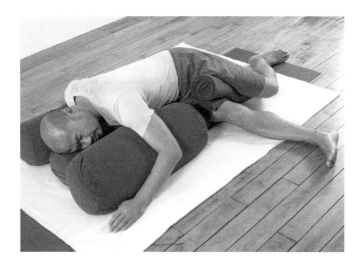

Props
Two blankets; three bolsters.

Timing
Same.

Alignment awareness

- Same.

- Actively straighten through the bottom leg while turning the abdomen across the middle line of the bolster and then resting the torso down. Relax the leg once in the posture. Note: the leg may bend slightly when resting into the pose; remember to adjust the grounded hip down away from the bottom of the bolster.

Anatomy and physiology

- Same.

- The arrangement of the bottom leg may be helpful for sciatic pain in this variation, creating more space in the outer hip joint and gently stretching the muscles along the outer buttock, hip and thigh.

Considerations, cautions and contraindications

- Same.

VARIATION 2: *ŪRDHVA MUKHA JAṬHARA PARIVARTANĀSANA*
Upward Facing Revolved Abdominal Posture with one leg straight.

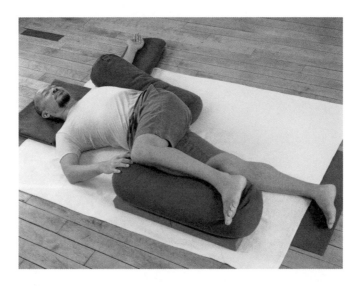

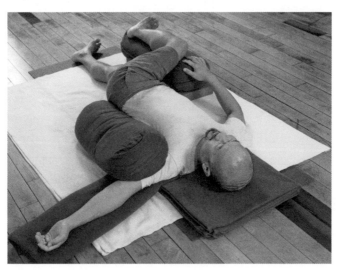

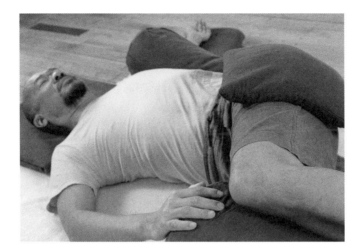

Props
Three blankets; two bolsters; two foam blocks; sandbag optional.

Timing
3–6 minutes.

Alignment awareness

- Start lying on the back with the knees bent. Shift the hips to the left away from the bolster/foam blocks placed to the right. Stretch the right leg down and then place the left knee, shin and foot over onto the bolster/ foam blocks. Allow the right foot to turn to the side. Stack the hips without forcing the placement. See that the bent knee is at a right angle and level with the outer top hip. Note: if the rotation causes discomfort in the lower back or the sacroiliac joints, raise the height of the knee, shin and foot to reduce the amount of rotation by adding/removing the foam blocks or an accordion folded blanket.

- Softly reach through the straight leg to anchor the spine; from this action lift the top of the chest and lengthen through the crown.

- Press the left hip down away from the head to lengthen the side of the waist and softly draw the top of the sacrum in so that there is a natural inward curve to the lower back.

- Optional: place a sandbag at the left hip and draw it slightly down away from the crown. Note: the sandbag can be placed this way in all variations.

- Place a bolster snugly into the back body (buckwheat is best) to lend support; pull the top of it up onto the front of the left shoulder to help ground it.

- Turn the top of the chest to face straight up towards the ceiling and lift the mid-sternum towards the chin while reaching the left arm out to the side. If needed, place an accordion folded blanket underneath the left arm and shoulder, especially to ground the back of the shoulder and arm if they do not easily reach the floor.

- Keep the head neutral with the back of the neck long, adjusting the height of the blanket so the forehead is a hair's breadth higher than the level of the chin.

- Briefly lift the head and look down the mid-line of the body to see if the nose, sternum and stacked hips line up. Adjust according to comfort.

Anatomy and physiology

- Same, apart from the shift from downwards to upwards.

- Broadens and opens the front body, allowing for a deeper breath into the lungs at the front and top.

- Front body opening tends to be more activating than its downward counterpart.

- Widens and spreads the clavicles, facilitating the opening of the thoracic inlet, which enhances lymphatic drainage back to the heart.

- Externally rotates and stretches the shoulder opposite the bent leg side and lifts the sternum, supporting an optimal postural re-alignment.

Considerations, cautions and contraindications

- For lower back or sacroiliac challenges – proceed with caution. Adjust the angle of the pelvis to alleviate discomfort by raising the support under the knee, shin and foot. Adjust the bolster supporting the back to include the sacrum. If there is still discomfort, avoid asymmetrical postures and rotation.

- For general discomfort or stiffness – consider more support underneath the shoulder and arm opposite the bent knee side and/or the shin to lessen the degree of rotation.

- For shoulder or neck discomfort – place the hand(s) on the front ribs bending the arm(s) to take weight off the shoulders. Support the elbows if needed. Consider adding support underneath the shoulders and the curve of the neck.

VARIATION 3: *ŪRDHVA MUKHA JAṬHARA PARIVARTANĀSANA*
Upward Facing Revolved Abdominal Posture with knees bent.

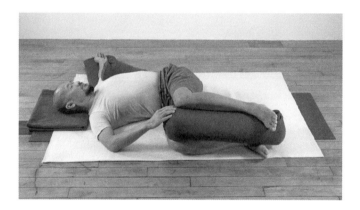

Props
Three blankets; two bolsters; foam blocks optional.

Timing
Same.

Alignment awareness

- Same, apart from entry into the posture, the arrangement of the legs (both knees are bent), and the bolster set-up (doesn't require foam blocks).

- Start lying on the side facing towards the bolster with both knees bent and at a right angle. Pull the bolster in between the knees, shins and feet. Press the right elbow into the floor to rotate the upper thoracic spine towards the left.

- Reach the left arm out to its side and rest it on the floor or an accordion folded blanket if needed. Note: two foam blocks can be placed underneath the right shin (essentially raising the floor) to minimize the depth of the rotation, if there is discomfort or the left arm doesn't easily reach the blanket.

Anatomy and physiology

- Same.

Considerations, cautions and contraindications

- Same.

SUMMARY OF POSE AND VARIATIONS

A twist or spinal rotation can be simultaneously invigorating, supporting fresh blood flow to the various tissues, and calming as it releases habitual patterns of holding. It opens up the rib area, encouraging depth and fullness of breath. The Restorative twist embodies transition as it adjusts the spine through its various expressions, serving as an intermediary between forward folding and back arches.

IV. Setubhanda sarvāṅgāsana
Classic Bridge Pose.

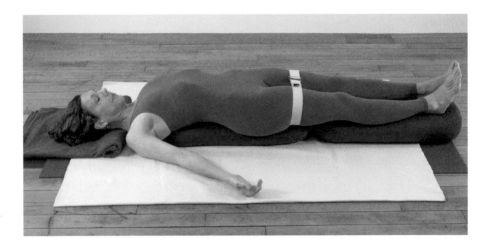

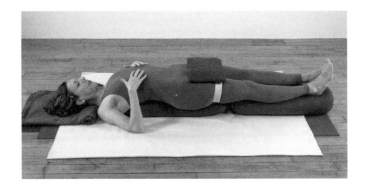

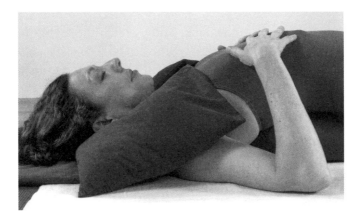

Props
Two bolsters; two blankets; one strap; sandbag(s) optional.

Timing
5–10 minutes.

Alignment awareness

- Place two bolsters end to end and sit towards the middle with the feet perched up on the bolsters. Tighten the strap around the mid-thigh so that the legs touch. It should be tight enough to keep the legs from rolling out, but not so tight as to cut off circulation.

- Lie back carefully with the knees bent. Slowly slide the torso along the bolster catching the skin of the back and the shoulder blades down until the top of shoulders reach the floor and feel grounded. The end of the bolster should rest at the back space of the heart, lifting the top of the chest. Note: if there is referred pain in the back, come further off the lift or swap out the bolster for accordion folded blankets 'stair-stepped' into the upper back to the height needed.

- Lengthen the neck spine adjusting up from the base of the skull. Soften the throat and relax the eyes. Avoid pushing the chin down.

- Optional: thinly roll a blanket to fit the curve of the neck spine. Do not raise the head up with the prop, rather just fit the blanket to the curve of the neck so that it is supported. Note: the addition of a rolled blanket to fit the neck curve for support can be made across all Restorative poses.

- If there is no pain in the back, softly stretch the legs down. Roll the thighs inwards and smooth the skin at the back of the pelvis down to prevent compression or discomfort in the lower back. Hook the inner heels towards the outer edge of the bolster. If discomfort arises in the lower back, work with the knees bent or lower the height of the lift.

- Optional: place a sandbag at the hip crease, grounding the top of the thighs, which helps release the spine. Place the sandbags at the top of the shoulders to ground the upper body and release the neck. Note: make sure the sand bags aren't pressing on the neck in such a way that restricts the flow of blood or the ability to breathe.

Anatomy and physiology

- Creates more physical space for the free and full function of the heart and lungs by opening the anterior chest.

- Widens and spreads the clavicles, facilitating the opening of the upper body.

- Tends to be more activating due to gentle extension of the upper back, which can stimulate the sympathetic chain.

- Decompresses the acromioclavicular and sternoclavicular joints.

- Externally rotates and stretches the shoulders, releases tension in the neck and upper back that can arise from a collapsed chest and forward head (sandbags help with this aspect).

- Helps relax the muscles at the base of the skull and in the face by supporting the curve of the neck, which promotes relaxation.

- Takes vertical weight off the spine, lessening disc compression and abdominal tension.

- Stretches the solar plexus, abdomen and diaphragm, releasing tension, which supports a deeper, fuller breath.

- Opens the space of the abdominal cavity, allowing perfusion of blood to the abdominal organs (versus constricted flow through compression).

- Is restful for the heart as it doesn't have to pump blood up against gravity to the brain.

- Gently stimulates the baroreflex via the baroreceptors in the carotid sinus in the neck, which has a quieting effect on the brain.

- Aids venous return to the heart with legs being level or slightly above the level of the heart.

- Holds the legs, via the placement of belt around the mid-thigh, allowing a sense of release that facilitates relaxation.

Considerations, cautions and contraindications

- Potential strain to the lower back and sacral areas – bend the knees or swap out the bolster for accordion folded blankets 'stair-stepped' into the upper back at a height that is comfortable.

- For neck pain or discomfort – adjust the support, which usually involves lowering the lift and/or supporting the neck with a rolled blanket to fit the curve of the cervical spine.

- Avoid the pose if there is eye pressure or retinal problems.

VARIATION 1: *SETUBHANDA SARVĀṄGĀSANA*
Bridge Pose with slightly elevated legs.

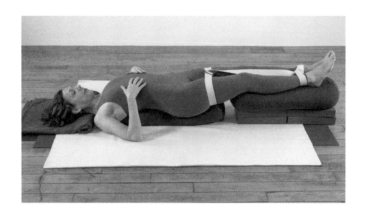

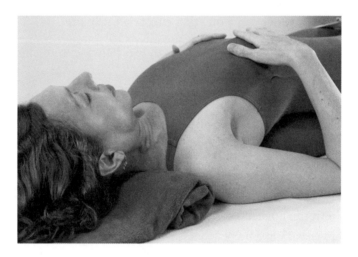

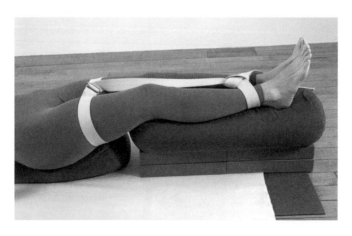

Props
Two bolsters; two blankets; four foam blocks; one strap.

Timing
Same.

Alignment awareness

- Same, with two layers of two foam blocks placed end to end underneath the bolster to raise its height. The raised legs can help with lower back discomfort.

- Consider tying the ankles with the tail end of the strap (or use another strap) for more support. Note: this strap adjustment can be applied to the classic version as well.

Anatomy and physiology

- Same.

- Further stimulates the baroreflex via the baroreceptors in the carotid sinus in the neck, which will have a quieting effect on the brain.

- Further aids venous return and the restful aspect of the heart, with legs being slightly above the heart, helping to prevent stroke and manage oedema.

Considerations, cautions and contraindications

- Same.

VARIATION 2: *SETUBHANDA SARVĀṄGĀSANA*

Bridge Pose with bolster placed widthways underneath pelvis and legs elevated onto a chair seat.

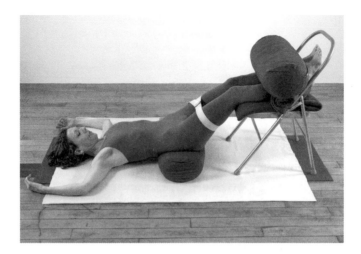

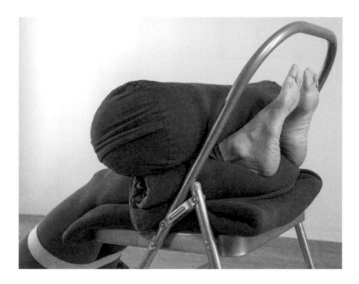

Props
Two bolsters; three blankets; one chair; one strap.

Timing
Same.

Alignment awareness

- Sit on a 'flattish' bolster placed widthways on the mat and face the chair seat. Swing the legs up onto the chair seat. Make sure the heels are supported by rolling a blanket underneath the curve of the achilles tendon. Note: for taller folks, consider using a second chair mirroring the first to support the heels.

- Optional: place a bolster horizontally across the shins for grounding.

- Position the strap at mid-thigh and hip width.

- Carefully lie back and make sure the bolster is underneath the sacrum, not in the lower back. Smooth the skin at the back of the pelvis down, anchoring the spine without losing the inward curve of the lower back. Note: the bolster should not increase the inward curve of the back.

- Remember to adjust the shoulder blades down the back, and lengthen up from the base of the skull.

- Reach the arms out to the sides and bend the elbows into a right angle – also known as 'cactus' arms. Turn the palms to face the head, resting the thumb-side of the hand on the floor. This helps create space across the top of the shoulder girdle.

Anatomy and physiology

- Same.

- Further stimulates the baroreflex via the baroreceptors in the carotid sinus in the neck, which will have a quieting effect on the brain.

- Further aids venous return and the restful aspect of the heart with legs being raised above the heart, which helps to prevent stroke and manage oedema.

Considerations, cautions and contraindications

- Same.

- For discomfort in the lower back or sacrum – remove the bolster underneath the pelvis and lie flat with the knees bent and calves on the chair seat.

VARIATION 3: *SETUBHANDA SARVĀṄGĀSANA*

Bridge Pose with bolster placed widthways underneath pelvis and feet on the floor.

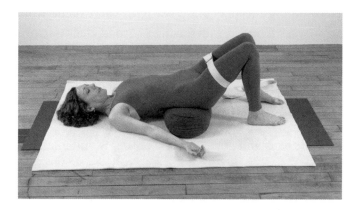

Props
One bolster; one blanket; one strap.

Timing
5–7 minutes.

Alignment awareness

- Same, with no chair.

- Place the feet flat on the floor and hip width apart; rest the thighs outwards into the support of the strap. Note: if the feet slide, fold the blanket back and place the feet directly on the sticky mat.

Anatomy and physiology

- Same, without 'further' stimulation of baroreflex and aid of venous return.

Considerations, cautions and contraindications

- Same.

SUMMARY OF POSE AND VARIATIONS

This pose has a calming and quieting effect on the nervous system that is also gently invigorating. The opening of the front body and gentle stretch of the back of the neck counter negative postural habits, releasing global patterns of tension. This mild inversion further stimulates the baroreflex, which has a deeply quieting effect on the nervous system that rejuvenates and revitalizes.

V. *Vīparita karaṇī*

The 'Practice of Inversion', also known as Legs up the Wall Pose.

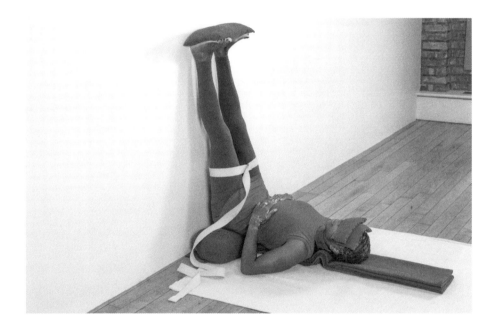

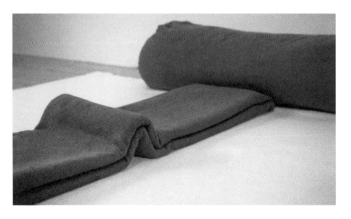

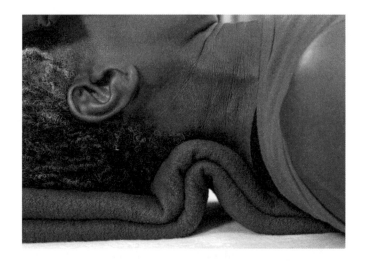

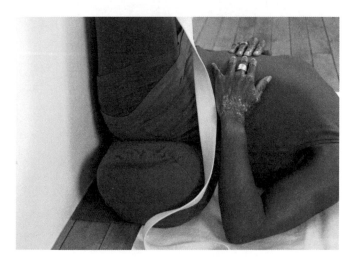

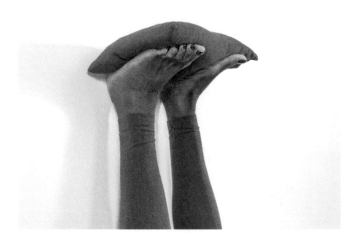

Props
One bolster; two blankets; strap(s) optional; sandbag optional; eye pillows optional.

Timing
5–10 minutes.

Alignment awareness

- Place a bolster horizontally on the mat about two to three inches away from the wall.

- Accordion fold a blanket from its long edge and place it perpendicular to and centred with the bolster. It should be long enough to accommodate the length of the torso and then some.

- Sit on the floor beside the bolster touching its end with the dominant hip; adjust the stance to feel the wall, lightly touching the back body. Position the feet to the side away from the bolster with the legs roughly in the shape of *bharadvājāsana*. Point the knees into the centre of the room away from the wall. Carefully lower the torso down using your dominant forearm for support, and roll the back of the pelvis up onto the bolster, swinging the legs up the wall.

- Bend the knees and press the feet into the wall in order to centre the pelvis on the bolster and the torso onto the blanket. Note: make sure the bolster is underneath the sacrum, not in the lower back. Ensure the blanket follows the spine.

- If possible, adjust the buttock bones to the wall. Release them downwards into the small gap between the bolster and the wall. Note: if there is a pulling sensation in the hamstrings, come further away from the wall and slightly bend the knees. In this situation, it's helpful to add support to the back of the thighs with bolsters or blankets to ground the back of the legs.

- Optional: place the strap mid-thigh if it helps create a sense of stability (i.e. being able to stay without holding or collapsing the legs). Note: add a second strap around the outer shins or ankles if it feels supportive.

- Optional: carefully place a sandbag on the feet by bending the knees; slowly straighten the legs, pressing the sandbag upwards, simultaneously softening the inner groin downwards. The sandbag adds a restful, grounding aspect that supports longevity in the pose.

- Adjust the shoulder blades down the back and lengthen the back of the neck. Make sure the whole of the back and head are supported on the blanket and that the skull doesn't end up on a seam or edge of the blanket (if so, come out and redo the accordion fold in the blanket to fit the whole of the torso and head). Make a small 'bump' in the blanket that seamlessly supports the inward curve of the neck. Re-adjust the base of the skull upwards.

- Place the hands on the front of the torso ensuring that the back of the arm and elbows are grounded or rest the arms at the sides away from the body with palms up.

- Note: if the wall is cold, consider wrapping the legs in a blanket. If the feet start tingling, bend the knees and place the feet on the wall.

Anatomy and physiology

- Due to the raised legs and pelvis, promotes a stronger baroreflex response via the baroreceptors in the carotid sinus in the neck, which has a deeply quieting effect on the brain.

- Assists the venous return of blood and lymphatic drainage from the lower part of the body through the raised legs, which helps prevent stroke and manage oedema.

- Takes vertical weight off the spine, lessening disc compression and abdominal tension.

- Creates space in the upper half of the abdomen/solar plexus, releasing tension in the rectus abdominus, obliques, transversus abdominus and linea alba.

- Relaxes and reduces in tension in the iliopsoas muscle. Widens and spreads the clavicles facilitating the opening of the thoracic inlet, which enhances lymphatic drainage back to the heart.

- Opens the chest, giving space to the thoracic cage and aiding cardiovascular and respiratory function by reducing compression on the organs.

- Releases tension in the muscles at the back of the neck, promoting health of tissue through haemodynamics.

- Releases tension in the neck, thus supporting a general sense of relaxation.

- Supports optimal postural alignment, especially when lying flat.

Considerations, cautions and contraindications

- If there is tingling in the feet – bend the knees and place the feet on the wall.

- For lower back or sacral discomfort – try lying flat with an even layer of cushioning underneath the whole of the torso.

- For tight hamstrings – come away from the wall and slightly bend the knees or place the calves on a chair seat with the knees bent.

- For menstruation – it's up to the individual with the guidance of a teacher/healthcare professional to choose what is appropriate and feels best. Lying flat with the legs up may be the most comfortable option.

- Avoid the pose if there is eye pressure or retinal problems.

- Avoid the pose if there is high blood pressure. A milder option would be to lie flat and bend the knees, resting the calves up on a chair seat.

VARIATION 1: *VĪPARITA KARAṆĪ*
The 'Practice of Inversion' with the legs crossed.

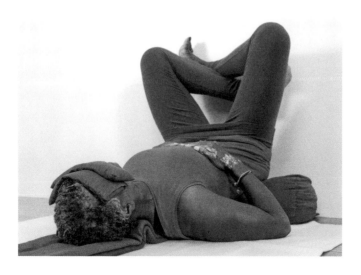

Props
One bolster; two blankets; eye pillows optional.

Timing
5–10 minutes – change cross of shins halfway through.

Alignment awareness

- Same, just bend knees and cross the shins. Note: if the wall is cold, place a blanket between the feet and the wall.

Anatomy and physiology

- Same.

Considerations, cautions and contraindications

- Same.

- Hamstring challenge may be alleviated through the bent knee variation.

VARIATION 2: *VĪPARITA KARAṆĪ*
The 'Practice of Inversion' without a wall and with a strap.

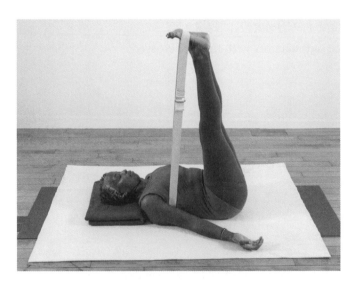

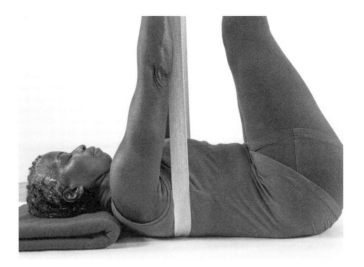

Props
Two blankets; one strap.

Timing
3–5 minutes.

Alignment awareness

- Make a big loop with the strap. First, place one end of the loop across the balls of the feet. Then, tuck the torso through the loop and place the other end of the loop at the tips of the shoulder blades. Note: do not allow the strap to slide down into the lumbar spine. The strap placement should facilitate the lift of the top of the chest.

- Organize the buckle so that it can be tightened/loosened with the dominant hand pulling towards the torso. Bend the knees slightly and loosen the strap a little. With resistance slowly straighten the legs towards a vertical placement while softening the groin back towards the floor keeping the pelvis grounded. There will be some muscular effort in this variation. If the hamstrings do not allow a straight leg, bend the knees so that the back of the pelvis rests evenly on the floor.

- If the strap cuts into the body or distorts the posture, loosen the strap and slightly bend the knees. Make sure the back of the pelvis remains on the ground. If it rolls up, loosen the strap.

- Pull the smooth edge of the blanket in to meet the top of the shoulders, so the neck and head are fully supported.

- Rest the arms by the sides with the palms up, or bend the elbows into a right angle into 'cactus'.

Anatomy and physiology

- Same.

- Stretches hamstrings and calf muscles.

- Takes the strain off the hands, wrist, elbows and shoulders, which is helpful for injuries to those areas.

Considerations, cautions and contraindications

- For tight hamstrings – bend the knees ensuring that the back of the pelvis stays grounded. If awkward, use the strap in the normal manner, holding the ends with both hands and dispensing with the loop.

SUMMARY OF POSE AND VARIATIONS
An ideal pose for 'putting the feet up' and taking a break. Helpful for those who spend long hours sitting or standing. This inversion stimulates the relaxation response and offers a deeply rejuvenating effect through the change in haemo-dynamics and internal pressure. It provides a restful way to re-align the spine.

VI. *Śavāsana*
Corpse Pose.

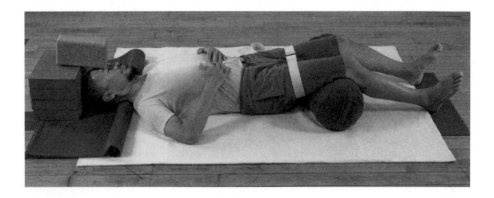

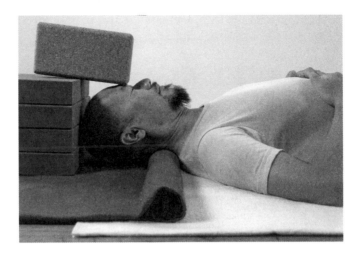

Props
One bolster; two blankets; one strap; four foams; one brick.

Timing
5–30 minutes.

Alignment awareness

- Place a bolster at the back of the knees to take the weight of the legs off the lower back spine, allowing it to soften.

- Secure the strap around the mid-thigh to hold the legs at hip width and parallel. Catch the thigh flesh inwards across the bolster to soften the groin, and place the belt snugly so that it keeps the legs from rolling outwards. Smooth the skin at the back of the pelvis downwards so that there is length in the lower back, and without removing the inward curve of the lower back spine. Sense the front of the pelvis narrowing, while the back of the pelvis widens and softens.

- Lengthen the achilles tendon by adjusting the heels away from the pelvis, and completely release the legs. For most people, the feet will turn slightly outwards against the constraint of the strap.

- Slide the shoulder blades softly down the back, lifting the top of the sternum upwards towards the throat. Fit a rolled blanket into the curve of the neck and adjust the base of the skull slightly upwards. If the forehead remains lower than the chin, increase the size of the rolled blanket and add another folded blanket underneath the head.

- Stack three or four foam blocks (depending on the width of the skull) just above the crown of the head. Position a cork/wood brick (lengthways/middle height) on top so that one end sits on the foam blocks and the other rests lightly at the space of the brow. The brick can be evenly placed or slightly adjusted downwards or upwards. If there is a lot of agitation, the downwards adjustment may be best to help settle the mind. If there is a lot of tension across the brow, the upward adjustment may be best to release the pattern of holding. In the end, try all three positions and see what feels best. Note: for the downward adjustment raise the height of the foam blocks a little; a light sandbag can also be used instead of the brick.

Anatomy and physiology

- Facilitates the complete and even relaxation of the body and whole nervous system.

- Supports optimal postural alignment in the torso.

- Relaxes the diaphragm, supporting easeful respiration.

- Removes the downward gravitational force on the intervertebral discs and the abdominal organs, which lessens disc compression and abdominal tension.

- Lessens the influence of gravity on haemodynamics – the heart doesn't have to pump blood up to the head against gravity and, similarly, the venous return from the legs and feet doesn't have to move upwards against gravity.

- Gently stimulates baroreceptors in the neck, triggering the baroreflex and quieting of the brain.

- Encourages the release of facial, neck and throat tension through optimal posture and head/neck support.

Considerations, cautions and contraindications

- For neck discomfort – fully support the neck and raise the head to suit the individual.

- For lower back challenges – use more support for the back of the knees. Other options to try are bending the knees as in Variation 1 or placing the calves up on a chair seat as in Variation 3.

VARIATION 1: *ŚAVĀSANA*
Corpse Pose with knees bent, also known as Effortless Rest Pose.

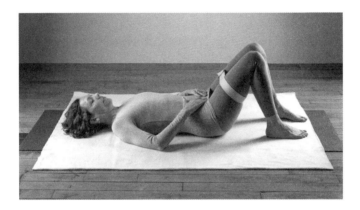

Props
One blanket; one strap.

Timing
5–15 minutes.

Alignment awareness

- Same, minus the bolster and with the feet placed flat on the floor with a strap supporting the thighs. This allows the lower back spine to soften into the floor.

- Comfortably place the feet hip width apart and parallel, and about a foot's distance away from the buttock bones – there is a sense of the thigh and shin bone resting in equilibrium against one another. The thighs are also placed hip width apart and rest into the support of the strap, which releases tension, particularly at the hips. Note: for some, resting the knees inwards against one another with the toes in and heels out offers a more comfortable option.

Anatomy and physiology

- Same.

Considerations, cautions and contraindications

- Same.

VARIATION 2: *ŚAVĀSANA*
Corpse Pose with legs elevated on bolsters placed widthways.

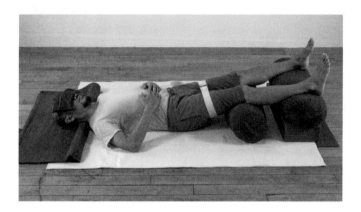

Props
Two bolsters; two blankets; one strap; four foams; eye pillows optional.

Timing
5–30 minutes.

Alignment awareness

- Same, with the addition of the props for elevating legs. Note: if you have enough props you may keep the brick on the forehead aspect.

- Rest the achilles tendon on the curve of the raised bolster placed widthways on four foam blocks, which serve as its base. Make sure that the whole of the bolster is supported so it doesn't tip, and that the heels are supported. If the feet dangle over the edge of the bolster, it will quickly become uncomfortable as gravity will pull on the unsupported parts of the body.

- Rest the backs of the knees on a bolster placed on its tall side, ensuring that there is plenty of support at the back of the knees.

Anatomy and physiology

- Same.

- Further stimulates the baroreflex via the baroreceptors in the carotid sinus in the neck, which will have a quieting effect on the brain.

- Further promotes venous return and the restful aspect of the heart, which helps prevent stroke and manage oedema.

Considerations, cautions and contraindications

- Same.

VARIATION 3: ŚAVĀSANA
Corpse Pose with legs on chair seat.

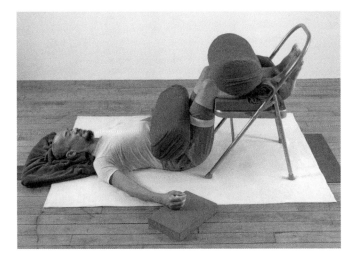

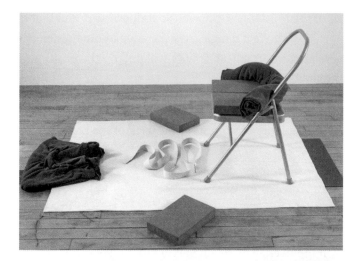

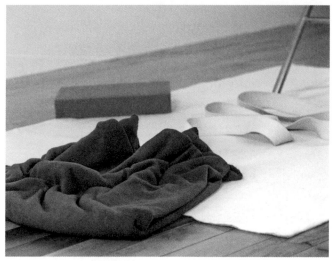

Props
Three blankets; one chair; one strap; two bolsters optional; four foams optional.

Timing
5–30 minutes.

Alignment awareness

- Swing the legs up onto the chair seat with the back of the knee at the edge. Note: place foam blocks or a blanket on the chair seat as needed so that the legs are set at a right angle. If the chair is too high for the length of the thigh, dispense with the chair and build a lift with bolsters to a suitable height.

- Make sure the heels are supported and not dangling. Place a rolled blanket under the achilles tendon to support the feet. Longer limbed folks may need a second chair mirroring the first, with the chair seat placed underneath the heels.

- Place a strap around the mid-thigh at hip width to prevent the legs from rolling out.

- Optional: place bolsters horizontally across the abdomen and shins for grounding.

- Optional: add a foam block under each hand aligning the wrist crease with the edge of the block. Especially useful for those whose hands do not easily rest on the floor, but hover just above it. Raising the hand onto the block grounds it, allowing the front of the shoulders to soften back and the neck to lengthen. Note: this adjustment can be used in any supine Restorative posture.

- Take a soft blanket and scrunch it up around the neck and the skull as a head cradle, making sure there is enough support underneath the head.

Anatomy and physiology

- Same.

- Releases tension in the lower back spine and across the sacrum.

Considerations, cautions and contraindications

- Same.

VARIATION 4: ŚAVĀSANA

Corpse Pose with torso elevated on an accordion folded blanket placed lengthways along the spine.

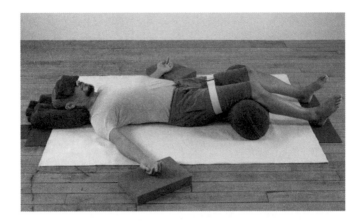

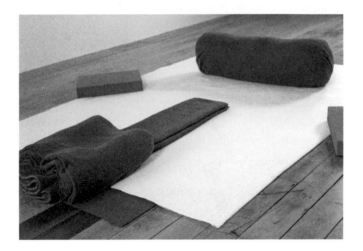

Props
One bolster; three blankets; one strap; two foams optional; eye pillows optional.

Timing
5–30 minutes.

Alignment awareness

- Same, without leg elevation and with added accordion folded blanket placed lengthways along the spine, and a blanket at the top cradling the head/neck.

- Sit in front of the blanket and carefully lie back so that the bottom edge of the blanket disappears into the lower back spine.

Anatomy and physiology

- Same, minus the inversion aspect.

- Gently extends the spine through the support of the blanket, opening the anterior chest and creating more anatomical space for the lungs and heart.

- Widens and spreads the clavicles, facilitating the opening of the thoracic inlet, which enhances lymphatic drainage back to the heart.

- Externally rotates and stretches the shoulders; opens the chest and lifts the sternum, supporting an optimal postural re-alignment.

- Relaxes the pre-cervical fascia and muscles of the throat, face, neck and shoulders, which supports relaxation.

Considerations, cautions and contraindications

- Same.

- For lower back challenges – remove the blanket, lie flat and use more support for the back of the knees. Consider bending the knees as in Variation 1 or placing the calves up on a chair seat, as in Variation 3.

VARIATION 5: *ŚAVĀSANA*
Corpse Pose with torso elevated on a bolster placed lengthways along the spine.

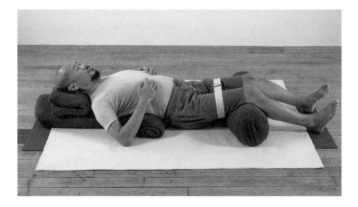

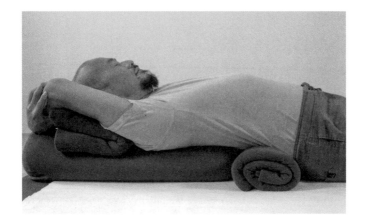

Props
Two bolsters; three blankets; one strap.

Timing
5–30 minutes.

Alignment awareness

- Same.

- In order to encourage the torso to release into the bolster, place a rolled blanket at the bottom to extend a gradual descending support for the spine.

- The arms can rest by the sides or place the hands on the front of the torso to facilitate breath awareness practices. When placing the arms, make sure the elbows and forearms remain supported.

- To increase the stretch of the shoulders and chest, which is helpful for breath awareness practices or transitions, take hold of the elbows with the finger pads and reach the arms over the head. Lengthen through the elbows so the sides of the trunk also lengthen. Do not force the arm/elbows down towards the floor. Do not hold the shoulder stretch overly long. Note: avoid this stretch if there is shoulder injury.

Anatomy and physiology

- Same.

Considerations, cautions and contraindications

- Same.

- For shoulder discomfort – place the hands on the front of the body and support the elbows. Do not reach the arms over the head.

VARIATION 6: *ADHO MUKHA ŚAVĀSANA*
Downward Facing Corpse Pose with widthways or lengthways bolster.

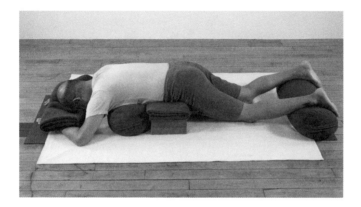

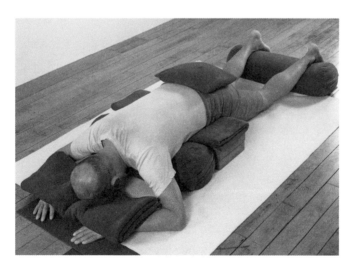

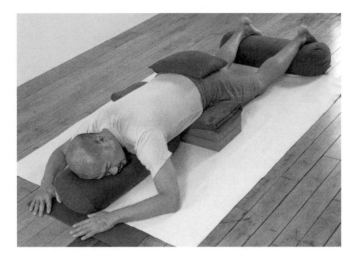

Props
Two bolsters; three blankets; four foams; sandbag optional.

Timing
5–30 minutes.

Alignment awareness

- Place a bolster widthways alongside a layer of four foam blocks padded with an accordion folded blanket to match the bolster's height. Position the hip creases at the bottom edge of the foam blocks/blanket and rest the torso downward facing, draped over the props. Note: you can turn the bolster 90 degrees placing it lengthways if this is more comfortable – in this variation, the head is turned to the side.

- Position a bolster at the hinge of the ankles. Allow the knees to rest down into the floor. Note: if the knees are sensitive, add more padding.

- Accordion fold a blanket and adjust it to fit into the curve of the forehead. Adjust the elbows outwards to release the shoulders. Alternatively, fold the arms back and support the front of the shoulders with blocks or blankets.

- Optional: place a sandbag at the tail. Gently pull it a little downwards towards the feet to anchor the spine.

Anatomy and physiology

- Same.

- Calms both physiologically and emotionally due to downward facing position; the protected sense of the front body encourages a feeling of safety.

- Promotes a quieting of the mind with the downwards orientation.

- Broadens the back body allowing for a deeper breath into the lungs (remember the lungs extend all the way to thoracic rib 10 at the back of the body).

- Reduces lordosis of the lumbar spine, gently stretching the lower back muscles.

Considerations, cautions and contraindications

- Some people may prefer lying on the back.

SUMMARY OF POSE AND VARIATIONS

The 'king' of the Restorative postures, *śavāsana*, removes fatigue, offering a deeply restful and rejuvenating period of time for balance, integration and assimilation. The evenness of its placement supports the quieting of the mind, fulfilling one of the goals of yoga practice. Every Restorative sequence includes a variation of *śavāsana* allowing ample time for rest and the practice of embodied presence.

Chapter 14

Sequencing

A journey transpires in a Restorative Yoga class with an apparent beginning, middle and end where a profound shift occurs in physiological state and perception. All this happens within the framework of time. Yet, each pose in a sequence represents an infinite moment in time – a powerful coming together of present moment awareness that is vibrant and spacious. So while there may be a sequence of poses, a coherent order that offers an intelligent progression, each *āsana* itself serves as an entry point into an ever-unfolding experience of fullness of being through embodied presence.

With this in mind, a Restorative pose can be practised on its own, or the postures can be sequenced for a complete practice. Restorative postures can also be added to a regular yoga class. I often start my yoga classes in *supta sukhāsana* – I find it a settling and softening way to formally begin – then gradually move into the more physical part of a class. Or, a Restorative pose can be well placed at the end of a more active sequence just before *śavāsana*. Restorative Yoga can be integrated in a way appropriate to the situation.

When crafting a Restorative sequence, it's important to think of context and the reasons for choosing this style of practice. At the beginning of a practice, the senses are outwards and the mind is active – there can be restlessness, tension in the body, stress or agitation. There may be tiredness captured in a 'forward moving' momentum, and the breath may be disturbed and unconscious. The energy at the beginning will reflect this through susurrant movement.

The arc of Restorative sequence allows for settling and a gradual inward turn of the senses. The timeframe and nature of the poses create the possibility for the body to relax from 'doing' and the mind from 'thinking'. The totality of a sequence enables the nervous system to move towards balance; the mind to

---

settle into equanimity; for there to be a tangible experience of space. The energy at the end of a class or pose will express the stillness of a relaxed, centred and grounded state.

PRINCIPLES
Set an intention and teaching focus
Craft an intention and teaching focus for the class/practice that creates coherence and determines its elements. Intention imbues meaning and purpose to action and provides the architecture on which a sequence hangs. A teaching focus establishes a specific learning point or awareness woven throughout the sequence that aligns with the intention. A clear intention and teaching focus drives the choice and order of postures and supports the spirit of learning and discovery within the totality of a class/practice. Begin with a pose that allows time to rest, settle and share the relevant aspects of the intention and teaching focus; always end with a variation of *śavāsana* that allows for assimilation, both understood and felt.

Choose simplicity
Once again, 'less is more'. Keep a sequence spacious, never ambitious. Allow time to slowly move from one pose to the next without urgency. Err on the side of fewer poses as transitions take longer, especially when the nervous system begins to quieten. Let simplicity serve as a guiding principle.

Include stretches
Include slow, supine stretches towards the beginning of a sequence that release physical tension in key areas to support the process of softening and opening. Stretches help bring more consciousness and awareness to the physical body – how it moves and feels. They provide a transition from outward to inward, allowing space to sense what is present; to settle into the gradually slowing pace of the sequence. It's here where restless energy can be dispersed, so that a pathway inwards can be established.

Incorporate breath awareness

Specific breath awareness exercises placed at the beginning of a sequence help settle the mind and shift the physiology. Breath awareness at this stage helps to establish the feel and texture of the body and cultivates the sense of the breath as 'teacher and friend'. It's here at this more alert stage of the practice that a softer, more conscious breath pattern can be cultivated, inspiring learning and discovery and forging a pathway inwards into the experience of embodied presence and essence.

Move from outward to inward

A sequence embodies a process of shifting from an outward orientation to an inward one. The first pose of a sequence, which can be held for longer to encourage settling and to establish the intention and teaching focus, encapsulates this transition. Slow, mindful stretches then follow to help release tension enabling a gradual transition to postures that are held for longer. This supports a slow and measured shift of state which allows for the practice of embodied presence towards the end, where stillness and silence reign. In this spirit, talking/instruction occurs more frequently at the beginning of a class and/or a pose to assist the move from outward to inward.

Hold poses for longer towards the end

The length of time held in a Restorative pose is determined by shape, action and placement in the sequence. Simple supine postures, such as variations of *śavāsana*, can be held the longest. Hold poses towards the end of a sequence for longer periods – the last pose (held for at least 10–15 minutes) allows time for deep rejuvenation without distraction, offering time for stillness, rest and the experience of embodied presence. Note: sometimes a sequence can incorporate a short meditation during a practice or end with meditation, or both. It's a matter of preference as to whether this happens before or after *śavāsana*.

Minimize and simplify transitions

Look at the sequence as a whole. Consider how to minimize and simplify transitions so as to create fewer disturbances. It's worth spending time looking at how prop arrangements can be repeated for different postures as a way to streamline the set-up and reduce movement and outer distractions. If a sequence uses a chair, pre-set the chair to avoid the disruption of having to get up and go get the chair.

Move the spine in all directions

Generally, a balanced Restorative class includes some kind of spinal extension, flexion and rotation, as well as an inversion in order to free the spine and help adjust the nervous system. This releases unnecessary tension and frees the breath. Avoid sequencing that keeps the body placed in one position (i.e. supine) for the whole sequence. Rather, vary the position and placement of the body in a way that moves the spine in all directions and prevents the discomfort that can arise when resting on a part of the body for too long.

Change directions of the spine with rotation or neutral

Always release the spine from either forward folding (flexion) or back arching (extension) with rotation or a posture that brings the spine back into its natural curves. For example, if starting a sequence with a supine posture that places the spine in a soft extension, rest in effortless rest pose for a short while afterwards. Then introduce either a supported or simple twist before shifting the direction of the spine into forward folding. This allows the muscles of the back to soften and work with the spine's change in direction.

Offer modifications and variations

Consider 'hot spots' in various postures (e.g. *bālāsana* – knees and ankles). Be prepared with adjustments, modifications and alternatives that address common challenges.

End with śavāsana

Every class includes some variation of *śavāsana* at the end of the sequence. This doesn't necessarily preclude its inclusion at the beginning. The king of all the Restorative postures, it's here where the deep work of balance writes itself into the nervous system, offering rejuvenation, resilience and wellbeing.

Allow time to reflect

Allowing time to reflect helps establish familiarity with the experience of balance and/or relaxation – how it feels, the sense of the nervous system in balance and so on. This is helpful for being able to recognize imbalance and make choices that help shift the physiology in the way that's needed. Observing the state of the body, mind and breath, particularly at the end of a sequence, helps to determine which kind of sequences work best. While outer factors may affect the end result, such as the state prior to the class/practice or the time of day, there can emerge a dominant feeling or energetic quality for a particular sequence which informs future choices and practices. Time for reflection can be built into the instruction through cues to 'observe' and 'notice'. This could also take the form of a formal meditation practice or writing in a journal.

FOUR SIMPLE SEQUENCES

Each sequence allows time in the first pose to establish a context for the class and engage with the intention and teaching focus – to encourage a settling inwards into the felt sense of the body and breath. Generally, stretches are best placed after the first pose; they can also be interspersed throughout the practice to help release tension and vary the texture of a sequence. A short, simple meditation can also be woven into the fabric of a class, in harmony with the intention and teaching focus. A sequence allows time for: demonstrating the set-up of each posture; articulating appropriate instruction; and spending time in stillness and space, especially towards the end of the sequence.

The timings of the poses include demonstration, setting up, instruction and stillness; the prop list reflects the set-up in the pictures.

Sequence 1

Intention: to promote evenness and calmness by encouraging the breath to flow with multi-directional ease.

Teaching focus: interrelationship between ribs and diaphragmatic movement.

Length: 1.25 hours.

Props: two to three blankets; three bolsters; two foam blocks; three cork bricks; one strap; eye pillow and sandbags optional.

Supta baddha koṇāsana: **Variation 2** (*supta sukhāsana*)
Reclining Easy Cross Legs Posture

20 minutes

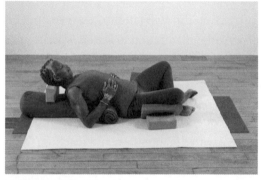

Adho mukha jaṭhara parivartanāsana
Downward Facing Revolved Abdominal Posture with bent knees to the right

9 minutes

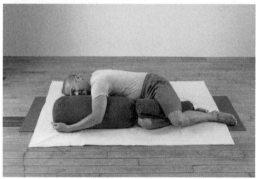

Balāsana
Classic Child's Pose

10 minutes

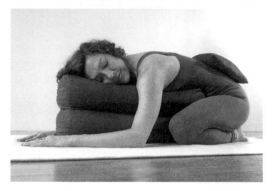

Adho mukha jaṭhara
parivartanāsana

Downward Facing Revolved
Abdominal Posture with bent knees
to the left

9 minutes

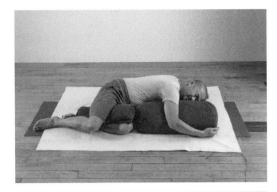

Setubhanda sarvāṅgāsana:
Variation 3

Bridge Pose with bolster placed
widthways underneath pelvis and feet
on the floor

7 minutes

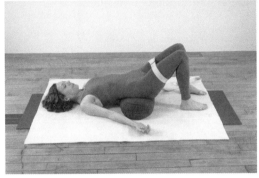

Śavāsana

Classic Corpse Pose

20 minutes

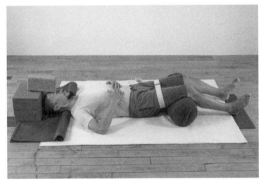

Sequence 2

Intention: to draw forth the mantle of wellbeing by engaging in a process of noticing, accepting and releasing patterns of holding through a free and easeful breath.

Teaching focus: identifying and working with patterns of holding.

Length: 1.25 hours.

Props: two to three blankets; two bolsters; four foam blocks; one strap; eye pillows and sandbag optional.

Śavāsana: **Variation 2**
Corpse Pose with legs elevated on bolsters placed widthways

25 minutes

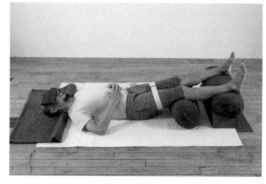

Vīparita karaṇī: **Variation 2**
The 'Practice of Inversion' without a wall and with a strap

5 minutes

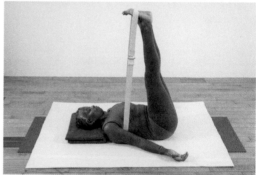

Ūrdhva mukha jaṭhara parivartanāsana: **Variation 2**
Upward Facing Revolved Abdominal Posture with one leg straight both sides

10 minutes

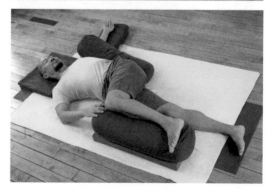

Adho mukha śavāsana: **Variation 6**

Downward Facing Corpse Pose with widthways or lengthways bolster

10 minutes

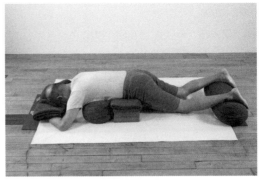

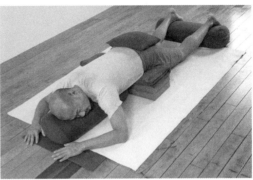

Short meditation

With focus on a free and easeful breath

5 minutes

Sit on foam blocks from previous pose

Śavāsana: **Variation 5**

Corpse Pose with torso elevated on a bolster

20 minutes

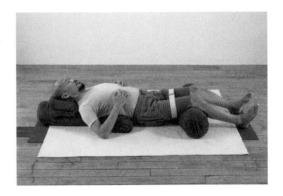

Sequence 3

Intention: to encourage slowing down and presence by learning how to extract the fullness of the present moment through the breath's expression.

Teaching focus: inhale-linger/exhale-linger.

Length: 1.25 hours.

Props: two to four blankets; two bolsters; two foam blocks; two cork bricks; one strap; eye pillow(s) and sandbag(s) optional.

Supta baddha koṇāsana
Reclining Bound Angle Posture with strap

20 minutes

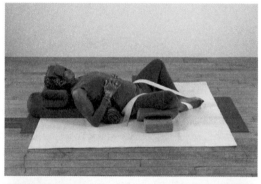

Śavāsana: **Variation 1**
Corpse Pose with knees bent, also known as Effortless Rest Pose

5 minutes

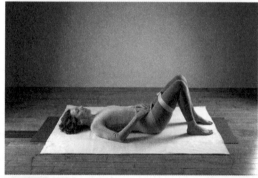

Stretches
Windscreen-wiper movement and thighs to chest

3 minutes

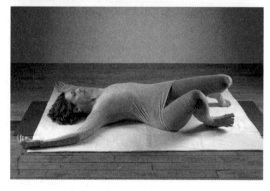

Balāsana: Variation 2

Child's Pose with the head down and bolsters placed lengthways with blanket across thighs

10 minutes

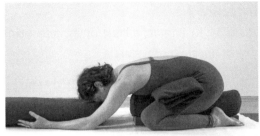

Short meditation

With focus on breath: inhale-linger/ exhale-linger

2 minutes

Stay seated on bolster

Setubhanda sarvāṅgāsana: Variation 2

Bridge Pose with bolster placed widthways underneath pelvis and legs elevated onto a chair seat

15 minutes

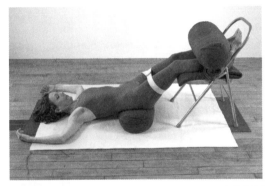

Śavāsana: Variation 3

Corpse Pose with legs on chair seat

15 minutes

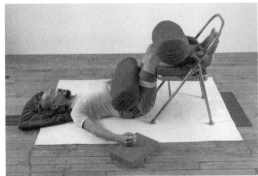

Meditation

With focus on breath: inhale-linger/ exhale-linger

5 minutes (or longer)

Sit on bolster or chair

Sequence 4

Intention: to support relaxation by cultivating the felt sense and raising awareness of physiological state.

Teaching focus: felt sensations of body and breath.

Length: 1.25 hours.

Props: two to three blankets; two bolsters; four foam blocks; one cork brick; one strap; eye pillow(s) and sandbag optional.

Śavāsana: Variation 4
Corpse Pose with torso elevated on an accordion folded blanket placed lengthways along the spine

20 minutes

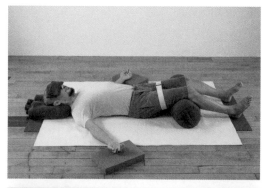

Śavāsana: Variation 1
Corpse Pose with knees bent, also known as Effortless Rest Pose

2 minutes

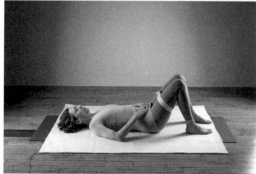

Stretches
Windscreen-wiper movement and thighs to chest

3 minutes

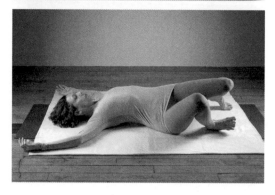

Balāsana: Variation 1
Child's Pose with the torso lifted
Turn head halfway through

9 minutes

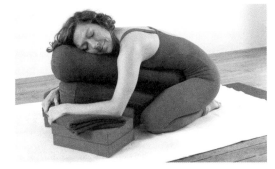

Vīparita karaṇī
The 'Practice of Inversion' also
known as Legs up the Wall Pose

8 minutes

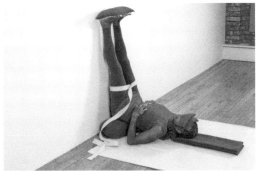

Vīparita karaṇī: Variation 1
The 'Practice of Inversion' with the
legs crossed
Change cross of legs halfway through

4 minutes

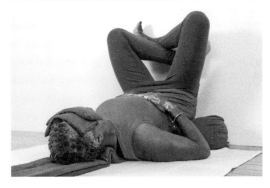

Meditation
Sensing body and breath

5 minutes

Seated on bolster at wall

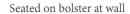

Śavāsana
Classic Corpse Pose

20 minutes

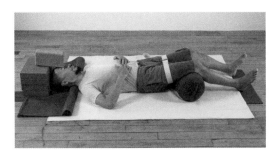

Chapter 15

The Art of Teaching
Restorative Yoga

CREATE A NURTURING SPACE

A Restorative practice or class becomes a sanctuary for experiencing space or stillness from the activities and speed of contemporary living. When creating a nurturing space, it's good to reflect a bit on general circumstances to understand the wider context within which the Restorative practice unfolds – transition from work, sitting all day, outer world developments, major life changes and so on.

It's best to assume that the stress of attending to the details and vicissitudes of daily life is written in the fabric of body and mind; that navigating the complexity of modern life leaves its signature in tension, perhaps overwhelm and fatigue. Coming to the mat may be the *only* time there is permission to let go and relax – a conscious choice to put on what Jean-Pierre Weill describes as, 'the hat and coat of wellbeing' (2013, p.54).[1] From the moment the decision is made to practice or come to class, a process of release can begin through conscious choice.

The art of teaching Restorative Yoga involves a number of different aspects that when combined offer a powerful way to help adjust the nervous system and move towards a state of balance that encourages the relaxation response. Everything from the arrangement of the physical space itself to the language of teaching and cues impacts the ability to 'switch off' and rest over the broad arc

---

1   This is a most amazing book and the illustrations are exquisite. His poetry encapsulates so beautifully the ethos and spirit of Restorative Yoga.

of a practice, setting the tone for 'being'. Since the primary intention of a class or practice is to encourage *a relaxed, grounded and centred state*, all choices with regard to the space, language and cues support the shift into a slower, more present state that aligns with this intention.

PRACTICE SPACE AS SANCTUARY

Sanctuary (noun) – 1. a holy or sacred place. 2. a building or room for religious worship. 3. a place that provides safety or protection... 4. the protection from danger or a difficult situation that is provided by a safe place... (Merriam-Webster online dictionary 2021).

The word sanctuary helps convey the ambiance of a space for Restorative practice that allows for its transformative experience, whether it's at home or in a studio. Much like a temple, the physical space itself supports a process for entering into the depths of being, the outer space being a reflection of the inner space. The way of entering the actual practice space can further enhance the movement towards balance and wellbeing.

During my years at the ashram, I learned about the importance of entering a sacred environment with reverence – from stepping into the space with the right foot forward and symbolically touching the heart, to walking through it with focus and presence in order to invoke an expansive inner experience. When beautifully arranged and pleasing to the eye, a sacred space can also generate a heartfelt movement towards connection.

The physical arrangement of a practice space or studio can radically support the shift of the physiology towards rest and the movement towards essence. I've had so many ideas of what an ideal Restorative practice space could look like. I'll share with you some that I've had... It's spacious and warm with heated floors; one end all windows revealing an expansive landscape of sky and beauty with mountains in the distance. It's a 'proper' retreat site dedicated to contemplative practice, nestled within nature; there are no disturbing sounds of city or humanity, just birdsong and perhaps the sound of burbling water – the sounds of Nature in her fullness. It would be fragranced with essential oils that are calming and pleasing, and fully stocked with a wide variety of props neatly arranged within an interior that speaks of spaciousness, warmth, beauty and simplicity. Perhaps take a moment and think of your ideal Restorative space...

What's recounted above points towards what's possible. My reality is that I'm usually in a small room in my house set up for yoga practice, a safe haven in the spirit of a retreat site. Your sanctuary may be your local studio, or the corner of the bedroom in your home situated in the busiest part of a city. Wherever you find sanctuary, take time to set up the space so that it's uncluttered, clean and inviting. Consider fresh flowers or some focal point to the space that inspires and uplifts. Cultivate a 'vibe' in the practice space that resonates with the focus of spiritual endeavour, that offers comfort and beauty, and provides a sense of protection. Set up a sanctuary for practice that invites the experience of relaxation and rest, setting the tone for self-enquiry, embodied presence and connection.

MOVE TOWARDS STILLNESS

I remember once a man coming up to me after a Restorative class in London. He thanked me for allowing silence in the practice space. He explained how he had attended yoga classes all over the world and was often frustrated because most yoga teachers talked through the *whole* practice, even in *śavāsana*. What he sought was space, *especially* in a yoga class, since the urban environments and situations he found himself in did not allow for stillness and presence. It's important to consider this aspect of 'sanctuary' – a place that serves as a refuge away from the stresses, talking and sounds of daily life – that allows for space, stillness and being.

With this awareness, most talking occurs at the *beginning* of the class while students are more alert and it's necessary to set the context, answer questions and prepare for the practice. In a similar way, most instruction and physical assists occur at the beginning of a pose, so there is undisturbed time and space in stillness. By the end of class or a posture, spaciousness resonates in the atmosphere; instruction and cues *if needed* emerge from an underlying blanket of quietude.

This raises the inevitable question about whether to play music or not – a choice that needs consideration. Playing music in a yoga class has become a new norm that has woven its way into modern yoga culture. Teacher trainings now offer this aspect as part of their curriculum (i.e. how to put a playlist together for class, positioning teachers as a kind of yoga DJ). While this may be popular and helpful for some to settle into a practice, I do not recommend playing music for Restorative Yoga out of respect for the transforming power of stillness, so much a part of its ethos. If it is felt that something is needed, choose something neutral and sparse that conveys the feeling of spacious presence.

VOICE AND BODY LANGUAGE

Tone of voice, content of instruction and body language play an extremely important role in creating a sense of 'sanctuary' that supports the relaxation response. When facilitating a Restorative practice, it helps when vocal tone is warm, modulates and is welcoming, accompanied by a smile. Again, in Porges' (2017) description of Polyvagal Theory, it is suggested that facial expression and vocal tone are intimately connected with feeling safe, and that prosody – the patterns of rhythm and sound in vocal tone – can reassure and comfort, supporting neural pathways for social engagement and relaxation. Being aware of this aspect can help guide the practice into relaxation and deeper states of being.

It's also helpful to explain a little bit at the beginning of a class about what to expect, giving some background about the style of practice and approach, and demystifying it. This means being clear with explanation and instruction as a way to help put people at ease, and know what they are supposed to do. Here are some things to consider with regard to voice and body language:

- *Be reassuring* – connect with students through gentle eye contact and a soft smile. Let a sense of ease and presence support the process of slowing down and connection.

- *Walk slowly and gracefully* – unhurried movement and slow gestures support a non-defensive response. While being quiet is important to support the atmosphere, avoid creeping up on people in a way that may startle them. At the same time, be aware of the weight of the step, so that the 'heel, ball, toe' roll of the foot is light.[2] Once the initial walking around to check set-ups is complete, come back to the teaching mat and stay present to the unfolding spaciousness, attentive to the needs of the students. Note: do not practise yoga yourself with the students while teaching. This distances the teacher/facilitator role and creates a disconnect that can be felt. Rather, be present and respond as necessary as the moment unfolds. I find sitting with eyes softly open works best.

---

2   At triyoga Camden in London there are beautiful wood floors from the time when the building was a factory. While the floors are lovely, there are parts that squeak in the most unappealing way! My assistant Sherman and I have learned over the years to avoid the squeaky bits, and once the initial adjustments are made, to promptly sit down wherever we are in the space so as not to disturb the emerging stillness. It makes for a rather interesting walking pattern.

- *Establish a methodical pace of instruction that modulates and explains –* take breaths in between cues so that instruction is easeful, can be heard, and use a normal, everyday voice. Speak naturally and clearly with a gentle intonation as in conversation with a friend. Avoid a monotone or putting on a 'meditation' voice. Let there be space in between instructions so that they land. Clarify instruction in a number of different ways to ensure understanding.

- *Use clear, simple language that invites enquiry and exploration –* craft invitational instruction which allows choice and reaffirms individual experience. Encourage students to make choices with regard to the set-up and practice that reinforce comfort, both physically and emotionally. While instruction allows for choice, it is also framed primarily in direct language or imperative voice, especially when it comes to setting up a pose. Clarity at this stage helps put students at ease. Repeat important alignment points and explain why. Once students are in a pose, your language of instruction can shift into a more reflective, invitational voice that supports inner exploration, enquiry and experience, allowing space for process.

- *Empower –* encourage exploration and choice so there is agency. While the shift to online teaching during the pandemic presented its challenges, it also created an empowered home practice environment. Students found themselves creatively improvising with makeshift props. I think this is beneficial as it encourages thinking about why a prop does what it does. An empowered stance invites learning and discovery which embraces the 'discipline' of practice as illuminating. Facilitating a class involves encouraging agency through informed choice, directly intervening only when it's absolutely necessary – if the set-up is incorrect in a way that could cause harm, or an assist could offer a deeper experience (as long as there is consent to touch).

PREPARING FOR THE PRACTICE

To be able to facilitate a nurturing class or practice, there are some aspects which can be attended to prior that help bring about the experience of sanctuary:

- *Get grounded* – arrive early and create a ritual or practice that grounds and centres in preparation for teaching or assisting a Restorative practice.

- *Refresh the practice space* – open windows if necessary and air the space. Sweep the floor. Make sure the props that are being used are clean and fresh.

- *Temperature* – allow ample time before the practice to close the windows if they are open, so that the space is warm. It's important that the room is a comfortable temperature. Body temperature can drop over the course of the practice, and being cold triggers a sympathetic response. Equally, a practice space that's too hot can also be uncomfortable. Ensure that the temperature supports balance and comfort.

- *Lighting* – become familiar with the lighting. It's ideal if the lights are on a dimmer, this way at the beginning of class or a pose, students can see. Over the course of a class or pose, the lights can be dimmed in order to support the relaxation response. By the end of a class, the lights can be switched off, as long as there is still some ambient light that allows safely exiting the practice space in the dark.

- *Sound* – make sure that extraneous sounds are minimal – close windows and consider the timing of a class in relation to other activities so there's not a clash. I remember once having a Restorative class while simultaneously a Rocket Yoga class was being held, which created a clash as the music accompanying the Rocket class intruded into the quiet space of the Restorative class.[3] I sometimes play tamboura, an Indian musical instrument often used for meditation, where the vibration of strings resonates in harmonious overtones that help minimize distracting sounds. (But this has its issues too, as it drives some students crazy!)

- *Pre-set the props* – this welcomes students into the practice and ensures that there are enough props for the planned sequence. It eliminates unnecessary movement and stress. It also allows for a late student to come in quietly without disturbing others in the shared space. A neatly arranged space with pre-set mats and props invites the student into the

---

3   It so happened in this case that the teacher involved was the lovely and bubbly Amme Poulton. While the actual situation created a conflict with regard to the approach of the classes, it gave rise to a sweet connection between us that endures to this day.

Restorative practice with the message that there is space for them and that they are welcome. Since experiencing space is integral to the Restorative experience, there ought to be ample space between students so the experience is both collective and individual.

- *Organize the assistants* – establish an 'assisting map' so that it's clear who is covering which area; this way people don't get over-assisted. It's helpful to establish 'home base', the place the assistant returns to after checking in with students at the beginning of a pose, and remains during the quiet parts of the practice.

ESTABLISH AN INTENTION AND TEACHING FOCUS

Preparing for the class involves crafting a sequence beforehand that arises from a clear overall intention and a specific teaching focus. Articulate this intention in some manner as people get settled into the first pose; touch on it throughout the practice supporting a focused and empowered learning environment based on discovery and self-care.

There are broad themes outlined in the text that follows that can serve as a source for crafting an intention/teaching focus, as well as help elucidate the purpose of Restorative Yoga. These themes touch on nervous system health and affirm balanced living. Note: keep the intention and teaching focus simple and non-proselytizing; remember, most talking occurs at the beginning of a class or a pose, allowing for understanding, exploration, choice and, finally, stillness.

- *Nervous system health* – since the Restorative practice is designed to shift the nervous system from 'fight or flight' to 'rest and digest', it's useful if people understand what helps support their nervous system in moving towards a state of balance and, eventually, relaxation. Pick one aspect below to work with as an intention/teaching focus:[4]

    - Encouraging a softer, more conscious breath which arises from the awareness of the diaphragm and is felt and followed.

---

4   It may be helpful to review 'Supporting the experience of relaxation' in Chapter 4, Nature of the Practice.

- Releasing unnecessary tension, emphasizing softening into the support of the props and gravity (focus on key areas of holding).

- Choosing comfort – which includes the set-up and temperature (i.e. cover with a blanket).

- Grounding and supporting the body.

- Feeling safe and cultivating a sense of sanctuary.

- Moving slowly and methodically with awareness.

- Pausing and savouring stillness.

- Holding poses for a period of time.

- Cultivating the felt sense.

- Supporting approach of investigation, acceptance and self-care, i.e. holding an intention to heal or move towards balance.

Sometimes it's helpful to use examples from everyday life for how we may (inadvertently) stimulate the nervous system:

- Reading emails before going to bed or first thing in the morning.

- Drinking too much tea or coffee, alcohol, eating sugary foods or smoking.

- Dwelling on things you have no control over.

- Obsessive or repetitive thinking about things of the past or future.

- Continuous activity without moments of stillness.

- Pushing yourself, especially when you are tired.

- Rushing.

- Unconscious, shallow or uneven breath.

- Stress brought about by major life changes/events.

- A perception of threat whether it's true or not.

- Focusing on news, stories, images or memories that evoke a strong feeling.

- *A free and easeful breath* – while every Restorative class ought to include some instruction that supports a free and easeful breath, it can also serve as the intention. The breath serves as a practical and empowering way to adjust physiological state. As the stress and habits of everyday life impact the breath through muscular tension, spend time exploring and releasing patterns of holding, particularly in the area of the diaphragm that may restrict its movement. Encourage the free movement of the diaphragm and explore how its pulsation moves the body — bones, muscles, organs and skin. Devise simple breath awareness exercises that support a free, efficient and easeful breath pattern.

- *Common areas of holding and releasing unnecessary tension* – Restorative Yoga offers a process for slowly letting go of muscular tension that can affect physiological state. Time can be spent scanning the body and observing where tension hides, then taking the support of the breath's movement to release it. Focus on common areas of holding and raising awareness; cue students to soften in these areas in relationship with the breath's natural movement (i.e. inhale – breathe softly into an area of holding; exhale – gently release unnecessary tension).

- *The power of present moment awareness and the felt sense* – encourage tuning in and feeling sensation as a way to stay anchored in the present moment and discern what is present – from the flow of the breath to the feel of the muscles and bones, sensations of coolness or warmth or sensing into deeper layers of the body and being. Use language that encourages and allows for unfolding experience – that gives permission to slow down and feel what is present (this also can include embracing outside noises that may occur as part of the moment).

  Affirm that emotions can sometimes arise during the course of practice, and are part of a process of release that is healthy. Leaning into and sensing the shape and texture of what is present, while attending the inner experience as a way to heal, forms an important aspect of Restorative practice. If the intensity of what is felt overwhelms, make it clear that it's fine to come out of a pose or even quietly leave the practice space (and come back) if needed.

  Placing hands on different parts of the body can help cultivate present moment awareness – the sensitivity and warmth of the hands grounds while supporting breath awareness as a way to feel and soften. The subtle awareness that can arise from experiencing, noticing and sensing the interrelationship between breath, body and mind, both internally and externally, sanctions innate wisdom and a sense of wholeness.

BEGINNING

Setting the right tone at the beginning of a class initiates a process of being able to lower defensive mechanisms and enter into a mode of being that reaffirms connection. While the general feel of a class is weighted towards silence, there are some points conveyed at the beginning of a class which orient and help students know what to expect. This undoubtedly supports a more restful and easeful experience. Note: some of the following points can also be addressed during the first pose.

- *Welcome people* – this can happen in a number of ways: helping people find a place as they come into the space; walking around and checking in with people; or formally introducing yourself at the beginning of the class and welcoming people to the practice.

- *Address newcomers* – ask who is new to the practice. This gives an idea of how much instruction may be needed and where to lend more support and encouragement. Let people know that you will talk more about the purpose of Restorative Yoga once they are settled in a posture.

- *Introduce the assistants* – if you have assistants (which is extremely helpful in a Restorative class), introduce them at the very beginning to establish their role as part of the practice. It also gives an opportunity to talk about assists; that if a student would prefer not be assisted, they can let the teacher and assistant know.[5]

- *Ask students to turn off phones and move personal possessions out of the way* – make sure that the sounds of phones do not disturb the quiet atmosphere, and the teacher and assistants do not step on something valuable or trip. This includes phones, water bottles (especially metal ones which clamour as they fall!) and bags. With regard to eye glasses, instruct the student to place them on a brick nearby, not on the floor. There is nothing worse than stepping on a student's glasses!

---

5   triyoga uses 'consent cards' that when placed on the mat indicate a student's choice with regard to being assisted, i.e. touched, which is helpful for teacher and student alike.

- *Discuss props, demonstration and the importance of comfort* – acknowledge the wide variety of props as a distinguishing characteristic of Restorative Yoga. Explain how the props support the body in the different poses, enabling longer holdings which help bring about the relaxation response. Note: for teaching online, clarify what people will need for the practice and address improvising with 'home' props.

  Unless you are teaching at a studio that emphasizes and trains in the use of props, most students won't really know how to use them. There may be anxiety around not knowing what to do. Explain that every pose will first be demonstrated, that there will be time to clarify the set-up, and settle comfortably into a pose. Reaffirm that comfort is an abiding principle for Restorative practice. Encourage students to adjust the set-up as needed or raise a hand for assistance; explain that adaptations and modifications for common challenges will be addressed for each pose.

- *Lighting* – mention that the lights will be dimmed once in the pose, and that by the end of the class there will be a period of time with the lights off. This helps students know what to expect.

- *Falling asleep* – because of adjustment to the nervous system, students can and do fall asleep. It's okay. This may be the very thing needed to address fatigue. The only time it becomes a problem is when people snore or breath heavily in a way that disturbs others. (Online teaching has solved the challenge of this aspect with the 'mute' button.) It's best to lightly address this at the beginning – that if this happens, the teacher/assistant will come around and place a hand lightly on their shoulder to make them aware – so they understand if this happens later. Normalize the situation at this stage, so they don't feel bad if it happens – it simply means they are starting to relax and this is good.

- *Leave worries at the door* – touch on the notion of sanctuary and highlight the importance of relaxation for health and wellbeing. Reinforce that it's okay to spend time in stillness and space; address in some manner implicit cultural assumptions that may interfere with the ability to pause and deeply rest.

DURING

- *Demonstrate the first pose of the sequence after briefly welcoming and orienting students* – call people around to observe the set-up. This can be a good time to talk about props and comfort and connect with people. It's the best time to invite questions and give clarifications, addressing modifications or alternative poses. Show how to fix the buckle on the strap and the best way to fold a blanket. If appropriate, demonstrate on a student or assistant. This allows for connection and ease in highlighting key areas that may pertain to the teaching focus or the set-up. It brings attention to the pose and props, rather than the personality of the teacher, deconstructing perceived differences with regard to the shape of the body and level of skill. If there are assistants present, demonstration helps clarify the set-up, and possible assists that relate to the teaching focus.

- *Allow time for students to set themselves up* – observe if they understood what was asked and then address common issues seen. Scan the room, helping first those who seem confused or uncertain and newcomers. In an unhurried manner, quietly walk the room to check if props are placed correctly, and that the students seem comfortable. Remember to smile and reassure, avoiding concentrated facial expressions that may be mis-interpreted. After a short while, return to the teaching mat and allow the students to settle. Guide them into an aligned posture with appropriate breath cues, re-establishing the intention/teaching focus for the class.

- *Demonstrate each pose in the sequence, allowing adequate time in each posture for stillness and space* – make sure instruction and assists do not disturb the inner experience of embodied presence towards the latter part of a pose.

- *Be aware of the rhythm of the class and adjust the lights appropriately* – after scanning and assisting the students at the beginning of a pose, dim the lights for the quiet part of the practice. Slowly raise the lights up (not too quickly) while bringing people out of a pose in preparation for the demonstration of the next pose. (An assistant can be very helpful in facilitating the transition of the lights.)

- *Encourage students to move slowly and methodically in between postures so as not to disturb the nervous system* – evenness in movement and tone help with this aspect. Sometimes a transition into the next pose doesn't necessarily require a demonstration, and may actually deter from the depth of the practice. It may also be the case towards the end of a sequence that physical adjustments and assists can be left out in order to support inner focus and quietude. Every class has its feel and rhythm – stay attuned to what's needed in the moment, making choices that move the practice towards stillness.

- *Pick poses in the final part of the sequence that can be held for longer and support rest* – as stillness becomes tangible in the space, both teacher and assistant become part of its fabric. Towards the end, students may fall asleep. It's at this moment that snoring can affect the experience of stillness in the communal space. It's incumbent on the teacher or assistant to gracefully handle this situation so that others aren't disturbed. Walk quietly to the student and gently place a hand on the shoulder, gradually adding more weight until they become aware. Hold your index finger to your lips (a universal quiet gesture), so the student immediately understands when their eyes flutter open in surprise. Having raised the point about snoring in the introduction of the class, this usually avoids a startled expression at its end!

AFTER

- *When the class ends, gradually turn the lights on* – as students start to move, ask students to move slowly and carefully, taking their time and letting their eyes adjust. Instruct students to put the props away neatly and with awareness so that it's part of the practice itself. Be available for questions, but at the same time encourage silence and stillness in the space, preserving the quiet energy of the practice.

- *Spend time after the class reflecting on your experience of teaching or assisting and consider what could improve the experience the next time* – each class adds to your knowledge of what works well and what doesn't and how to better support people in their experience and practice of Restorative Yoga.

ASSISTING AND THE POWER OF TOUCH

'Assisting' someone during a Restorative practice not only nurtures through the power of touch and care, it helps refine the placement of the body in such a way that can make all the difference to the experience. An 'assist' in Restorative Yoga involves physically adjusting the body through touch or a prop in order to render a pose more easeful and comfortable. Discerning what's needed and adapting a set-up in the least obtrusive way represents an integral and skilful part of teaching and assisting Restorative Yoga.

- *An assist or adjustment represents an integrating action that supports natural movement and healthy alignment, and reinforces nervous system balance and wellbeing* – an assist or adjustment can be verbal, a gesture, demonstrated or involve touch as well as props. Sometimes offering an assist can be viewed as trying to 'fix' people. It's best to avoid framing an assist in this way, which implies that a student is doing something wrong or is lacking in some way, or that the teacher is the sole holder of knowledge. Remember, an assist or adjustment is offered in collaboration with a student in order to make a pose feel more comfortable and to aid the relaxation response. It empowers a student by *offering* applied knowledge through direct experience. This lends itself to making informed choices with regard to future practices. An assist also conveys what is meant by 'easeful' and 'restful', and establishes a frame of reference that can be drawn on not only in practice, but in everyday life.

- *The environment of a class provides sanctuary, and what this means to an individual can vary widely* – for some people, receiving an assist may be the only time they are engaged with or touched. Increased isolation and loneliness, lack of nurturing contact or trauma will impact the choice and approach of an assist. For some it's a welcome and needed aspect, while for others it's an action that can illicit fear and extreme suffering. A class or practice offers a way to positively connect with others – whether through an assist, a smile or in sharing a collective practice space – that supports feeling safe and at ease in order to relax.

- *Establish consent before assisting or adjusting a student* – by addressing assisting at the beginning of a class, it makes it easier to check in with a student before adjusting them in a specific pose. Offer an assist or adjustment at the beginning of a pose when a student is more alert and can make their wishes known. A clear demonstration that explains the set-up and offers alternatives also helps to minimize the need for an adjustment that requires direct touch. If there is a situation where the student doesn't wish to be adjusted, and the set-up may be injurious, ask the student to make the assist/adjustment themselves and explain why. Note: an online context adds another level of sensitivity to the aspect of offering an assist. It can be jarring to be called out by name in an online class, especially in Restorative Yoga. Rather, offer encouragement and acknowledgement first. Then, if needed, be specific about adjusting the set-up to be more comfortable, and invite the student to try it if they want, so it's not about having done something wrong.

- *Ensure the student can hear the teacher/assistant approach to avoid startling them* – while being quiet in manner and bearing is important to the overall atmosphere of a class, a little bit of rustling or the sound of approach/activity helps a student orient to the location of the teacher and/or assistant and this can be reassuring.

- *Kneel to the side of a student before making an assist to check in and be at the same level* – if an adjustment requires standing over the student for its safe application, again ask if this is okay. Standing over a student can be intimidating; it can completely undo the efforts made to ensure a student feels safe, which defeats the wider purpose of the practice.

- *Having gained consent, remember to smile and connect with the student, offering the adjustment with presence, respect and sensitivity* – when making contact, touch should be firm, reassuring and gentle. Never force the body in a direction it doesn't want to go. Consider the simplest and most effective way to make the adjustment you need to make with the least amount of disturbance. Minimize talking and use gestures when possible. Make the adjustment in an unhurried manner, but at the same time don't linger. While there may be an impulse to comfort, simply apply the assist in a way that is neutral, yet kind and compassionate, remembering that an adjustment represents a shared effort and process that moves towards a state of comfort, ease and connection.

- *Apply assists/adjustments according to need* – attend first to newcomers and those who look confused or may hurt themselves if they stay in the pose. Then, methodically work through the room checking set-ups.

Avoid singling out a particular person. Stay sensitive to the moment when it's time to stop, and allow the room to settle into stillness.

- *Different bodies may require a different set-up, i.e. more or fewer props* – while there is a recommended set-up of props presented in the demonstration, one size does not necessarily fit all. When assessing a pose, consider the foundation first and then look at the overall shape of the student in the pose. Assess if the student looks comfortable, and if the props are appropriately supporting the body. Consider if another prop or set-up may be better. For example, swapping out a firm and round bolster for accordion folded blankets offers a lower, flatter base which may be a better choice, even if it means the student has to get up. If you change the props, check in with the student, and make sure that they are comfortable with the change. Have a back-up pose in mind if the one that is being explored doesn't work for the student – keep it simple and easy.

  The final placement in a Restorative pose is guided by each student's unique situation and comfort level. Help students find the most optimal alignment possible in their body, using an assist/prop to provide the alignment or action in the body that may be missing.

- *Make sure the body is supported as much as possible* – sometimes it may be pulling the blanket more snugly into the back of the neck, and under the head. Or placing a blanket underneath an elbow or the hands. Sometimes it can be the small, innocuous adjustments that make a world of difference.

And, finally, if assisting a Restorative class, watch what assists/adjustments the teacher gives and follow suit. Minimize verbal adjustments for the sake of quiet. Stay sensitive to when the teacher stops assisting, indicating it's time to settle and become still. The assistant acts like an extra pair of hands for the teacher. To reiterate, most assists occur at the beginning of the pose; allow time and space for stillness and silence at the end of pose, and the end of the class.

Chapter 16

Experiences of Restorative Yoga

It's been a time of reflection, and taking stock of what I am able to offer to others. This is actually what I believe practice has been for me – the continued renewal, balance and reflection of how I am performing for myself, and for those around me. Without the discipline of my practices, the clarity they enable, life can become a challenge, which can easily tip the other way. On the flip side, with practice and perseverance, all these challenges become something that I feel willing to embrace – as another great opportunity to strengthen both my character and the deep relationships that I am blessed to share with those around me. So my everyday practice is how to embrace life (practice makes perfect?). For me Restorative Yoga makes sense; it has been, and continues to be, the most rewarding study.

I still clearly recall being in class with my legs up against the wall. Anna suggested that next time rather than drinking a coffee, I should try lying with my legs up the wall for ten minutes, and then see if I still felt the need for coffee… This has really stuck with me. For me, it's an excellent reflection. Those moments where, if we allow it, we could easily step up our output for the sake of keeping up with the requests of others. At these times, rather, just taking that brief moment to pause, consider and then respond is so very valuable. In this 'legs up the wall' moment, a lot of clarity can come…

Actually practising recovering and restoring has been one of the most beneficial practices I have come to embrace after that first legs up the wall moment. From my previous balance of energy it was clear that intense physical and mental output would burn – and were burning – me out. Investing time

---

and effort in learning the tools which can enable restoration, and better balance, gifted me a second wind. Thank you!

Andy Beyst
Holistic fitness consultant

I respond to the rhythm of Restorative Yoga. When we start slowing down, intentionally placing the props that will support us and reclining onto the mat, I feel ready to let go of the concerns of the day. I gently place an eye pillow over my eyes so they can rest, as it's likely I have been looking at a screen or text for too many hours.

These rituals allow the mind to begin to settle and come into the body. As our practice begins, I feel able to release and start to experience my grounded presence.

I relish the stillness as the body opens into the intended release of the *āsana*. The *āsanas* that are designed to give the spine more support or focused stretch bring great comfort.

Several years ago, I developed lower back problems and Restorative practice is a key support that I use to avoid lower back pain and maintain flexibility overall. When we are in an *āsana* designed to give the body a gentle twist, I feel a nourishing release that I do not find easy to access through other physical activities. During the practice from time to time, we are guided to notice the breath and explore and deepen it. As I rest in the pose, the breath is present, but there is no effort to engage with it or direct it, such as when practising *prāṇāyāma*, and this natural breath is more relaxing.

I really savour the expanse of time in the practice and the pleasant rhythm of being suspended in a pose for some time, and eventually making a gentle transition into another *āsana* for an alternative form of release. For me, Restorative practice provides a crucial way to quiet the mind and fully inhabit my body. As time slows and suspends, I am able to rest in the present moment, which allows some precious opportunities to experience the unfolding of boundless consciousness.

I find the practice both a form of and a perfect segue into meditation, which is my main spiritual practice. I was first exposed to meditation practices of Buddhist and Hindu traditions on a gap year to South and South-East Asia nearly three decades ago. I was a member of a Hindu spiritual community for over 20 years and also studied with Mahayana Buddhist nuns for five years. I came to Hatha Yoga later on and have been practising Restorative Yoga for 17 years now.

Restorative Yoga is a wonderful companion to sitting meditation. Often after a class finishes I take a few more minutes to stay and sit in meditation and find I am able to reside in the stillness and go deeper. By that point my nervous system has been calmed by the practice and I don't experience the usual kinds of disturbances that might greet me when I sit down to meditate. My thinking mind is very quiet and able to rest within a nurtured body. Gravitating towards the stillness of Restorative Yoga is a cherished way for me to maintain my wellbeing and connection with spirit.

Felicity Daly
Academic and yoga practitioner

I have regularly practised different forms of yoga for the last 15 years, but have found Restorative Yoga to be the most transformational practice for me. I had my first encounter with Restorative Yoga when I was taking my final exams at university. I had become so stressed and overwhelmed that it was inhibiting my wellbeing and academic performance. I tried Restorative Yoga and it was such a healing experience. Although I had known about the benefits of yoga on an intellectual level, by practising yoga at a time when I really needed help, it created a deep experiential understanding of its benefits, which created a profound trust in the process. It is trust that when life becomes overwhelming, there is always a place to rest and restore on the yoga mat. Restorative Yoga has provided me with a powerful antidote to the feeling of stress in daily life ever since.

At times, my practice has slipped because I am a naturally busy person who has more tasks than I can fit into a day. It is easy to fall into the mentality of 'once I have done everything I need to do, I can relax'. But this moment never comes. Instead, the busy momentum that I create for myself only accelerates, leaving me with less and less time to practise. Not only this, but I find that when I do then come to the mat, it is more challenging and takes a longer time to access that space within me where my tension melts away and my mind quietens.

But the deep trust that I have in the process always brings me back to the mat. It is by staying still and allowing myself to actively engage with the process of conscious and deliberate relaxation that I get to access it quicker and with greater ease over time. Over the years, I have found that Restorative Yoga has become one of my top priorities regardless of what is going on in my life. This is because, previously I had practised in response to stress I was experiencing in order to help reduce it and restore my sense of balance and inner peace. I was practising in reaction to something; to help calm me down so that I could carry on. But then I experienced a deeper appreciation for it when I began to regularly practise. I found that the benefits I experienced on the mat were better able to be carried off the mat and be with me in everyday life. The more I practised shifting states – shifting from the fast-paced demands of daily life to the quiet calm on the mat – the more I was able to shift states quickly and respond to stress in real time by breathing through it and allowing it to pass through me rather than sticking to me. It felt like having muscle memory, where every cell in my body had learned how to let go and relax. So when I needed to call on this tool, it was readily available to me without too much effort. One of the further benefits I was able to carry off the mat is that I became better able to stop giving such a deep narrative to what I was experiencing, and just experience it. It helped me stay present.

Taking the lessons practised on the mat into my life is where I feel that Restorative Yoga has benefited me the most. Having recently gone through a painful and challenging life experience, I found that my ability to stay present, breathe, let go of unnecessary narratives and physically release tension allowed me to be less reactive and generally more able to cope. This peaceful place that I am able to access through Restorative Yoga has become a comfort and a coping mechanism that I would recommend to anyone. Especially if Anna is your teacher!

Jodie Jackson
Author and founder of Little Ruffle

I have turned to Restorative practice in many different ways over the years; carving out big chunks of the day to practise for a few hours, taking a posture or two in between teaching classes to restore energy levels, starting an Ashtanga practice and ending up cocooned by blankets. And when some may have opted for a siesta, I have headed to my mat for *upaviṣṭha koṇāsana* or the like. I have dreamt of planes where instead of seats everyone was given bolsters and blankets, and we could all travel in *supta baddha koṇāsana.*

It's fair to say that this practice has made a huge impact on my life, but it is often difficult to express this in words. So, when Anna asked me if I would write a few words on why I practise Restorative Yoga, I felt a need to roll out my mat, take a posture and just lean into the experience once more. As human beings we always wish to repeat good experiences, so what exactly is it that keeps me coming back for more, and with a strong desire to share this practice with others? As I lay over the bolster two words came to mind: quietening and nourishing.

As I am someone who wakes up early and is active for much of the day, it creates the space for me to think less and feel more and be, rather than do. While some people may choose to play music during their Restorative practice, for me this practice is about exploring the silence and stillness. In the beginning, it is all about the physical body; finding comfort so that I can relax and be still. Staying in position allows me to feel where I am holding tension, and how my body softens and releases it. With the physical body in place, I become aware of my body breathing; the flow of energy begins to change and my mind gently quietens. After a few minutes, I drop down into a feeling of spaciousness and ease. In deep relaxation, you hover in a place where you are neither asleep nor fully awake, and the mind naturally quietens. Resting in this spaciousness, you become free of everything; there is no physical body, no mind and certainly no emails to be dealt with!

Of course, there are days when it is difficult to settle into the practice; the body can't find comfort in the postures, and the mind keeps pulling us out. I have experienced many practices like this over the years, and frequently at the beginning of the pandemic of 2020. For me, these practices are insightful; while everything on the surface appears fine and you keep telling yourself and others that everything is fine, the practice is telling a different story. It's often an opportunity to look at what changes need to be made both on and off the mat. In the case of the pandemic, lots of things were out of our control, but just continually returning to the grounding nature of the practice and enjoying moments of deep rest, as brief as they sometimes were, was invaluable. Restorative practice was a wonderful coping mechanism for a stressful situation, and provided a chance to step back and rest in a safe and familiar place.

After practice, I leave the mat with my feet firmly on the floor but with a lightness in my physical body. I feel well rested, with a clear mind, and the tasks that felt onerous before the practice feel more manageable. Nourished by the Restorative practice, I find a sense of calm pervades and I am ready to interact with the world outside again.

Joyce McMiken
Restorative Yoga teacher

Restorative Yoga has been a revelation for me. I've been practising it in classes and on retreats for around seven years.

With all the craziness of the city, Restorative Yoga with Anna at triyoga in London has been an oasis. I so often went to a class buzzed up and racing in my mind to the next adrenaline hit awaiting me. Sometimes it would take five minutes; sometimes half the class, but, inevitably, I would find peace. The peace manifested in my body as I surrendered to the postures; in my mind as it slowed right down; and in my breath where I would often observe that the rhythm of my breathing had changed without any conscious effort. Another unexpected side effect was that on the days I was practising Restorative Yoga, my sleep pattern changed. It usually became easier to drop off and the relentless monkey mind felt tamed.

Prior to discovering Restorative Yoga, I had seen yoga as a kind of workout with the added bonus of spiritual connection. Now, Restorative has become my most loved form of yoga practice.

It has been said that the best way to still the mind is to move the body. And this has also proved true with Restorative Yoga. Although I have practised meditation for decades, some of my sweetest moments of serenity have come unbidden while holding the gentle poses inherent in this form of yoga. I love the fact that all the poses are stress free and invite me to truly relax every bone, every muscle and every breath in my body.

I am now in my seventies. In my thirties, the vigour of Ashtanga would have spoken much more to me, but there are hidden depths in Restorative that my younger self would have ignored. If my body is going to continue being a reliable vehicle for my life, then Restorative Yoga is a blessing, and its subtlety like a sweet wind on a hot day.

Thank you, Anna, for being a true embodiment of this practice and an outstanding teacher and inspirer.

Malcolm Stern
Psychotherapist, author and co-founder of Alternative

Restorative Yoga has given me a sense of coming home to my body and myself. Through it I experience a kind of rest that is unlike any other and feels deeply healing. There is physical and emotional release and mental calming. As I relax into the poses, I'm aware of my digestive system working properly; my heart feeling at rest; my breathing soft, even and deeply pleasurable; and my mind free from rumination and anxiety. It is odd perhaps that something apparently so simple as relaxing can produce such profound effects. But I feel that Restorative Yoga heals on all levels, and challenges the strange assumption of our culture that we need to strive and suffer in order to gain any benefit from a physical discipline.

Sarah Deco
Teacher of Tai Chi Movements for Wellbeing, and storyteller

I discovered Restorative Yoga in 2007 and it's been a major part of my life since then.

I had been attending Anna's Hatha Yoga classes at triyoga in London, and noticed at the end of class that most people weren't leaving. Anna was asking people to add another bolster and two blankets to their collection of props (for what I now know was the Restorative class following her Hatha Yoga class).

The next week I too stayed on after Hatha and literally floated out of the Restorative class. Why? The stillness and support of the Restorative practice resonated with me; it provided me with space to reconnect to myself. The use of props provides the support and the room is dimly lit and at an ambient temperature. All these factors allow my nervous system to know I'm safe and shift from sympathetic to parasympathetic mode, relaxation. Homage to Mr Iyengar for his creation of both the props and the practice of Restorative Yoga.

Restorative Yoga became part of my regular practice and today, being honest, I practise (and teach) more Restorative than Hatha Yoga. This is probably because Restorative Yoga has helped me navigate some difficult phases in life, allowing me reduce my stress levels and keep grounded, and provided space to rest when I was pushing twice as hard as a black woman to be seen in the corporate world and dealing with the micro-aggressions that unfortunately are a part of my life.

Restorative Yoga provides me with an opportunity to reconnect to my breath, to pause, to see myself more clearly as the stillness and quiet allows me to release any tension and when the tension is released the magical relaxation can be allowed in. At the end of a Restorative practice there is a definite increase in my sense of calm and wellbeing.

I teach Restorative Yoga because I want to share the benefits I have had from the practice over many years with others. Plus, I genuinely believe that society could do more to promote the importance of pause. That said, I believe the pandemic has helped people to slow down a bit more and realize what is important to them.

I love giving students the opportunity to pause, rest and reconnect with themselves, lessening their stress and anxiety levels. Restorative Yoga allows people to navigate life a little more easily; I feel that I am providing students with a vital item to add to their toolkit for life. I love hearing the varying positive comments after a Restorative class from some students feeling so relaxed it's an effort to move or speak; feeling as if their bodies are screaming thank you and clearing mind blocks to allow progress.

I am thankful for the day I met Anna and discovered Restorative Yoga, a truly healing part of my life.

Yvonne O'Garro
Restorative and Hatha Yoga teacher

SUMMARY OF PART III
Regular practice of Restorative Yoga realizes a 'new' definition of discipline which embodies a process of deep investigation and learning, and invites the lived experience of balance. Practice as a wellspring imbues teaching with power and presence. Through postures which nurture and sequencing which allows time and space in stillness, this practice offers sanctuary. The art of teaching Restorative Yoga facilitates a transformative experience held by practitioner and teacher alike, which adjusts physiological state, supporting the relaxation response and sowing the seeds of connection vital for wellbeing.

References

Ackerley, R., Badre, G. and Olausson, H. (2015) 'Positive effects of a weighted blanket on insomnia.' *Journal of Sleep and Medicine Disorders*, 2(3), 1022.

Antonovsky, A. (1987) *Unraveling the Mystery of Health: How People Manage Stress and Stay Well*. San Francisco, CA: Jossey-Bass.

Barnhart, R.K. (ed.) (1988) *The Chambers Dictionary of Etymology*. Edinburgh: Chambers Publishing.

Bateson, G. (1979) *Mind and Nature: A Necessary Unity*. New York, NY: E.P. Dutton.

Bateson, N. (2016) *Small Arcs of Larger Circles: Framing Through Other Patterns*. Axminster: Triarchy Press.

Benson, H. and Klipper, M.Z. (1975) *The Relaxation Response*. New York, NY: William Morrow & Company.

Bernard, C. (1974) with translations by Hoff, H.E., Guillemin, R. and Guillemin, L. *Lectures on the Phenomena Common to Animals and Plants*. Springfield, IL: Charles C Thomas.

Birch, J. (2011) 'The meaning of *haṭha* in early haṭhayoga.' *Journal of the American Oriental Society*, 131(4), 527–554.

Bryant, E.F. (2009) *The Yoga Sūtras of Patañjali, A New Edition, Translation, and Commentary*. New York, NY: North Point Press, a division of Farrar, Straus and Giroux.

Calais-Germain, B. (2006) *Anatomy of Breathing*. Seattle, WA: Eastland Press.

Cameron, J. (1992) *The Artist's Way: A Spiritual Path to Higher Creativity*. New York, NY: Tarcher/Putnam Book, G.P. Putnam's Sons.

Cannon, W. (1932) *The Wisdom of the Body*. New York, NY: Norton.

Cantor, D. and Ramsden, E. (eds) (2014) *Stress, Shock, and Adaptation in the Twentieth Century*. New York, NY: University of Rochester Press.

Cope, S. (2012) *The Great Work of Your Life: A Guide for the Journey to Your True Calling*. New York, NY: Bantam Books, an imprint of Random House, a division of Penguin Random House LLC.

Davidson, R.J. *et. al.* (2008) 'Regulation of the neural circuitry of emotion by compassion meditation: Effects of meditative expertise.' *PLOS ONE*, 3(3), e1897.

Eliot, T.S. (2001 [original work published in 1944]) *Four Quartets*. London: Faber and Faber.

Feuerstein, G. (1998) *Tantra: The Path of Ecstasy*. Boston, MA: Shambhala Publications.

Grimes, J. (1996) *A Concise Dictionary of Indian Philosophy, Sanskrit Terms Defined in English*. Albany, NY: State University of New York Press.

Iyengar, B.K.S. (2012) *Body is My First Prop*. Pune: Ramāmaṇi Iyengar Memorial Yoga Institute.

Iyengar, B.K.S., Evans, J.J. and Carlton Abrams, D. (2005) *Light on Life: The Yoga Journey to Wholeness, Inner Peace and Ultimate Freedom*. Emmaus, PA: Rodale Books.

Kempton, S. (2011) *Meditation for the Love of It: Enjoying Your Own Deepest Experience*. Boulder, CO: Sounds True.

Koolhaas, J.M. *et al.* (2011) 'Stress revisited: A critical evaluation of the stress concept.' *Neuroscience and Biobehavioral Reviews*, 35(5), 1291–1301.

Kuvalayananda, S. (ed.) (1926) 'Śavāsana or the Dead Pose.' *Yoga-Mimamsa*, 2(3), 229–232.

Labour Force Survey with Health and Safety Executive (2020) *Work-Related Stress, Anxiety or Depression Statistics in Great Britain, 2020. Annual Statistics*. London: HSE.

Lakshman Joo, S. (2007 [second edition]) with translations by Baumer, B. *Vijñāna Bhairava Tantra. The Practice of Centring Awareness*. Varanasi: Indica Books.

Lasater, J. (1995) *Relax and Renew: Restful Yoga for Stressful Time*. Berkeley, CA: Rodmell Press.

Li, Y. and Owyang, C. (2003) 'Musings on the wanderer: What's new in our understanding of vago-vagal reflexes? V. Remodeling of vagus and enteric neural circuitry after vagal injury.' *American Journal of Physiology. Gastrointestinal and Liver Physiology*, 285(3), G461–G469.

Mahony, B. (2014 [second edition]) *Exquisite Love*. Davidson, NC: Sarvabhāva Press.

Mallinson, J. and Singleton, M. (2017) *The Roots of Yoga*. London: Penguin, Random House.

Merriam-Webster (2021) Merriam-Webster.com Dictionary. Springfield, MA: Merriam-Webster. Accessed on 22/04/21 at www.merriam-webster.com/dictionary/presence; accessed on 22/04/21 at www.merriam-webster.com/dictionary/prop; accessed on 22/04/21 at www.merriam-webster.com/dictionary/sanctuary.

Morris, J. (2020) *The Unwinding and Other Dreamings*. London: Unbound Press, United Authors Publishing.

Moyer, D. (2006) *Yoga: Awakening the Inner Body*. Berkeley, CA: Rodmell Press.

Muacevic, A. and Adler, J.R. (2018) 'The influence of breathing on the central nervous system.' *Cureus*, 10, 6, conclusion.

Nixon, P.G. (1982) 'The Human Function Curve – A paradigm for our times.' *Activitas Nervosa Superior*, 3(1), 130–133.

Olivelle, P. (2008) *Upaniṣads, A New Translation*. Oxford: Oxford University Press.

Porges, S. (2011) *The Polyvagal Theory: Neurophysiological Foundations of Emotions, Attachment, Communication, and Self-Regulation*. New York, NY: W.W. Norton & Co.

Porges, S. (2017) *The Pocket Guide to the Polyvagal Theory*. New York, NY: W.W. Norton & Co.

Porges, S. (2020) *The Neuroscience of Polarisation*. Rebel Wisdom. Accessed on 22/04/21 at https://rebelwisdom.co.uk/films/13-film-content/science-and-psychology-of-polarisation/580-dr-stephen-porges-the-neuroscience-of-polarisation-pt-2-of-4.

Powell, S. (2018) *The Ancient Yoga Strap: A Brief History of the Yogapaṭṭa*. The Luminescent. Accessed on 22/04/21 at www.theluminescent.org/2018/06/the-ancient-yoga-strap-yogapatta.html.

Rosen, R. (2002) *The Yoga of Breath: A Step-by-Step Guide to Pranayama*. Boston, MA: Shambhala Publications.

Rosen, R. (2017) *Yoga FAQ: Almost Everything You Need to Know About Yoga from Asana to Yama*. Boston, MA: Shambhala Publications.

Rosenberg, S. (2017) *Accessing the Healing Power of the Vagus Nerve*. Berkeley, CA: North Atlantic Books.

Selye, H. (1936) 'A syndrome produced by diverse nocuous agents.' *Nature*, 138(3479), 32.

Selye, H. (1946) 'The general adaptation syndrome and the diseases of adaptation.' *Journal of Clinical Endocrinology and Metabolism*, 6(2), 119–131.

Selye, H. (1974) *Stress Without Distress*. Philadelphia, PA: Lippincott Williams & Wilkins.

Shantananda, S. (2003) *The Splendor of Recognition*. South Fallsburg, NY: SYDA Foundation.

Singleton, M. (2010) *Yoga Body: The Origins of Modern Postural Practice*. New York, NY: Oxford University Press.

Singleton, M. and Goldberg, E. (eds) (2014) *Gurus of Modern Yoga*. New York, NY: Oxford University Press.

Sundaram, Y. (1928) *The Secret of Happiness or Yogic Physical Culture*. Coimbatore: The Yoga Publishing House.

Swātmārāma, S. (2002) with English translation by Akers, B.D. *The Hatha Yoga Pradipika*. Woodstock, NY: YogaVidya.com.

van der Kolk, B. (2014) *The Body Keeps the Score*. London: Penguin, Random House.

VanderWeele, T.J. (2020) 'Activities for flourishing: An evidence-based guide.' *Journal of Positive Psychology & Wellbeing*, 4(1), 79–91.

Vimuktananda, S., translation (2019) *Aparokṣānabhūti attributed to Sri Śaṇkarācārya*. Kolkata: Advaita Ashram. Accessed on 22/04/21 at http://yogananda.com.au/upa/Aparokshanubhuti/aparokshanubhuti_01.html.

Wallis, C.D. (2013 [second edition]) *Tantra Illuminated: The Philosophy, History, and Practice of a Timeless Tradition*. Petaluma: Mattamayūra Press.

Weill, J. (2013) *The Well of Being*. New York, NY: Flatiron Books.

Wheatley, M.J. (2017) *Who Do We Choose To Be? Facing Reality, Claiming Leadership, Restoring Sanity*. Oakland, CA: Berrett-Koehler Publishers.

Wheatley, M.J. (2018) *Warriors For The Human Spirit*. Colorado: Sounds True. Accessed on 22/04/21 at www.resources.soundstrue.com/transcript/margaret-wheatley-warriors-forthe-human-spirit.

Yogendra, S. (1928) *Yoga Asanas Simplified*. Mumbai: The Yoga Institute.

Further Reading

Essential Help for your Nerves: Recover from Nervous Fatigue and Overcome Stress and Fear, Dr Claire Weekes (1984 [revised edition 2000])

Evolving Your Yoga: Ten Principles for Enlightened Practice, Barrie Risman (2019)

Original Yoga: Rediscovering Traditional Practices of Hatha Yoga, Richard Rosen (2012)

Resonate with Stillness, Gurumayi Chidvilasananda (1995)

Somatics: Reawakening the Mind's Control of Movement, Flexibility, and Health, Thomas Hanna (1988)

Stitches: A Handbook on Meaning, Hope, and Repair, Anne Lamott (2014)

The Balance Within: The Science Connecting Health and Emotions, Esther M. Sternberg, MD (2001)

The Blue Zones: 9 Lessons for Living Longer, Dan Buettner (2008 [second edition 2012])

The Book of Joy: Lasting Happiness in a Changing World, His Holiness the Dalai Lama and Archbishop Desmond Tutu with Douglas Abrams (2016)

The Breathing Book: Good Health and Vitality Through Essential Breath Work, Donna Farhi (1996)

The Gift: Poems by Hafiz The Great Sufi Master, Daniel Ladinsky (1999)

The Power of Now: A Guide to Spiritual Enlightenment, Eckhart Tolle (1999, 2005)

The Whole Body Breathing: Discovering the Subtle Rhythms of Yoga, Sandra Sabatini and Michael Havkin (2018)

The Wisdom of Insecurity: A Message for an Age of Anxiety, Alan W. Watts (1951 [second edition 2011])

The Yoga of Discipline, Gurumayi Chidvilasananda (1996)

Waking the Tiger: Healing Trauma, Peter Levine with Ann Frederick (1997)

Wherever You Go, There You Are, Jon Kabat-Zinn (1994)

Why Zebras Don't Get Ulcers: The Acclaimed Guide to Stress, Stress-Related Diseases, and Coping, Robert M. Sapolsky (1994 [third edition 2004])

Index

Note: Page numbers to illustrations are given in *italics*